Praise for

THE VITALITY MAP

"Deborah Zucker is a gifted healer, working with great compassion to help others find their holistic health mojo. Her book will be a beacon and a gift to many."

—ELIZABETH GILBERT, author of *Eat, Pray, Love*

"Health involves more than a normal physical exam, blood tests, and scans. 'Health' is related to 'wholeness' and 'holy'—how we fit into the grand pattern of existence, where we find meaning, purpose, and fulfillment. Dr. Deborah Zucker is a wise guide who will help anyone go beyond the 'merely material' to find what genuine health is all about."

—LARRY DOSSEY, MD, author of *One Mind*

"*The Vitality Map* reveals the path you need to take to find your true self and fulfill your meaningful desires and needs. Deborah's words are a guidebook and life coach on your journey through life."

—BERNIE SIEGEL, MD, author of
The Art of Healing and *365 Prescriptions for the Soul*

"Deborah Zucker offers a foundational piece missing in our urgency to 'get better': a skillful and compassionate relationship with the process of healing ourselves so that our illnesses can become gateways to a more integrated life."

—VICKI ROBIN, author of
Blessing the Hands that Feed Us and *Your Money or Your Life*

"Dr. Deborah Zucker offers an excellent traveler's guide for authentic self-care that reanimates you at all levels of your being. She takes you on an intimate journey into these deeper realms of self-care, effortlessly weaving together a wide array of methods—psychotherapy, spirituality, physical health, and community—into one integrated approach. *The Vitality Map* shines light on what really matters in life and inspires you to become deeply healthy so that you can bring your best self forward in all that you do. I am inspired by the contribution that Dr. Deborah Zucker offers in this important work to the field of medicine as a whole. May her message be heard and give us all the courage to live with more vitality!"

—BARON SHORT, MD, MS, Brain Stimulation Service Medical Director, Associate Professor at Medical University of South Carolina

"*The Vitality Map* will guide you through a more vital and holistic approach to your health and reveal to you the hidden treasures of a balanced way to eat, nurture, and care for yourself. Deborah is a magical health guide that will lead you on your journey to optimal health! Keep this book by your side!"

—AGAPI STASSINOPOULOS, author of *Unbinding the Heart*

"In an era of dramatic change and constant stress, maintaining your health is more challenging and also more imperative than ever before. In her new book, Dr. Deborah Zucker beautifully interweaves the principles of spirituality and health to offer a robust and novel approach to addressing health challenges. *The Vitality Map* provides useful tools to develop both physically and spiritually, and shows you how awakening to deep health makes possible the fullest realization of your own potential."

—MAUREEN METCALF, CEO Metcalf & Associates, Inc. and author of the *Innovative Leadership* Workbook Series

"Most of us are more worried about disease, but what we need to turn our attention to is optimum health and vibrant vitality! Deborah Zucker has a 'get real' conversation with the reader on one of the most pressing issues of the maniacal modern day—how to get back their inner mojo, motivation, and momentum. With her 9 keys to wellness, she makes the path to becoming vital illuminating and enlightening, even when we feel like we are in the dark and burnt out with no hope left. Follow her great beacon of wisdom!"

—DEANNA MINICH, PhD, author of *Whole Detox*

"This book is a gem. True healing necessitates more than visiting the doctor, taking the medication, staying on the diet, or doing the exercises. How we find the wholeness and empowerment within ourselves is vital, and Dr. Deborah Zucker has designed a clear and engaging guide for recognizing and reclaiming greater vibrancy and health. A valuable resource to engage with and savor!"

—LUANN OVERMYER, author of *Ortho-Bionomy: A Path to Self-Care*

"Deborah Zucker invites you on a sacred journey to your own healing potential which brings you into intimate contact with your inner wisdom and beauty. Each step along the way is rooted in self-compassion, gratitude, and trust in yourself. *The Vitality Map* points the way to who you've been looking for."

—JANETTI MAROTTA, PhD, author of *50 Mindful Steps to Self-Esteem*

"*The Vitality Map* is the essential guide for growing your health. Dr. Deborah Zucker ushers us into the depths of our aliveness and provides unparalleled instruction on how we can holistically approach vitality and well-being. This extraordinary work instills compassion, illuminates much needed clarity, and touches our human vulnerabilities with grace. *The Vitality Map* is the new path forward and we all have a responsibility to follow Dr. Zucker's wisdom."

—ROB MCNAMARA, author of *The Elegant Self* and *Strength to Awaken*

"Whether you face health challenges or wish to maintain your current health status, *The Vitality Map* is a wonderful guide to ensuring that you have covered all bases. So many of us obsess over our 'numbers' on test results, or believe that taking our daily pills is the maximum expected of us to ensure our health. But it is far from the truth. We now understand that the body/mind/spirit connection must be factored into our daily regimen. Consider this book for yourself or for a friend with health challenges."

—LYNNE D. FELDMAN, MA, JD, author of *Integral Healing*

"Every individual body, imbalance, and healing process is unique. Yet the shape of the hero's journey of restoring health can be charted. And the practical know-how of navigating the detective work and practice of healing can be described. Dr. Deborah Zucker has traveled this path, and this book shares the wisdom, savvy and tips she's learned navigating her own healing and in guiding others as a health practitioner. This lonely journey just got a little less lonely."

—TERRY PATTEN, author of *Integral Life Practice*

"Dr. Zucker provides your personalized roadmap to freedom, health, and happiness. Embracing the feminine, the shadow, and bringing in her rich experience as a mind-body-spirit provider, I have yet to encounter a more insightful, well-crafted, and helpful book."

—GEORGIA TETLOW, MD, CEO of Philadelphia Integrative Medicine and Assistant Professor of Rehabilitation Medicine, Thomas Jefferson University

"When it comes to creating health and well-being in our lives, most of us have very good intentions. We just fall short in the follow through. Dr. Deborah Zucker's book, *The Vitality Map*, gets to the root of why we so often fail and gives us a path to true and lasting success. You have to go deep and *The Vitality Map* takes you there."

—BONNIE HORRIGAN, author of *The Bravewell Story* and Editorial Director of *EXPLORE: The Journal of Science and Healing*

"I am honored to join the growing list of supporters for Dr. Deborah Zucker's new book, *The Vitality Map*. Her experience and teachings are clear, guided messages that will enlighten the mind, heart and spirit. The honest word here is DEEP; no hype or fluff in this world of quick fixes. Dr. Zucker's 9 keys are most relevant for anyone who seeks lasting peace, health, and the vitality needed for a deeper, more meaningful life."

—JO ANN STAUGAARD-JONES, author of *The Vital Psoas Muscle* and *The Concise Book of Yoga Anatomy*

"Dr. Zucker manages to go way beyond current spiritual and medical paradigms without violently shredding those ideas to pieces as I've too often seen. She truly has stood upon the shoulders of giants with grace and has offered a logical, doable system for healing and for living our greatest potential. By incorporating the strengths of both the left and right brain and inviting us to viscerally embody her time-tested ideas through various recommendations and exercises, a new road map of healing and wholeness has become clear. I believe this will be a best seller for years to come!"

—DAVE MARKOWITZ, medical intuitive
and author of *Self-Care for the Self-Aware*

"At least 97% of Americans lack one or more of the essentials for health. And at least 90% of illnesses are the result of poor health habits! *The Vitality Map* offers the guide to optimal health!"

—C. NORMAN SHEALY, MD, PHD,
Founder and CEO International Institute of Holistic Medicine

"Deborah Zucker is a profound healer who helps people discover their own potential for maximum health and growth. Her book *The Vitality Map*, with its 9 Keys to Deep Vitality, provides not just theories, but tested tools and proven strategies for whole-person healing. This remarkable book can truly unlock the mystery of integrated body, mind, and spirit wellness and should be a trusted guidebook for everyone who desires optimum health."

—KAREN WYATT, MD, author of *What Really Matters*

THE
VITALITY MAP

A GUIDE TO DEEP HEALTH, JOYFUL SELF-CARE, AND RESILIENT WELL-BEING

DR. DEBORAH ZUCKER

LomaSerena
PRESS

2016

The author of this book does not dispense medical advice or prescribe the use of any technique as a form of treatment for physical, emotional, or medical problems without the advice of a physician, either directly or indirectly. The intent of the author is only to offer information of a general nature to help you in your quest for physical, emotional, and spiritual well-being. In the event you use any of the information in this book for yourself, the author and the publisher assume no responsibility for your actions.

Contact:
LomaSerena Press
info@lomaserenapress.com

Ordering Information:
Special discounts are available on quantity purchases by corporations, associations, and others. For details, contact the publisher at the address above.

Cover and interior book design: Claudine Mansour Design

First Edition, May 2016

Paperback ISBN: 978-0-9974089-1-1
Digital ISBN: 978-0-9974089-2-8

Printed in the United States of America

CONTENTS

ACKNOWLEDGMENTS

THERE IS NO WAY that I could have written and birthed this book without the tremendous support of the incredible communities, colleagues, clients, and loved ones that make up the web of connection in my life. This book may have come through me, but it was born from all of you.

I feel so deeply blessed by the unconditional loving support of my parents, Sharon and Elliot Zucker, whose generosity and unerring belief in me held me as I navigated the healing journey that I share in these pages. You have both made it possible for me to develop, nurture, and express my unique gifts—it is because of this support that Vital Medicine exists and that I was able to write this book. You have always wanted me to align with what brings me vitally alive and to authentically share what I am here in this life to share. You, dear Mom and Dad, are the best!

A big hug and acknowledgment of gratitude goes to my brother, Jonathan Zucker. It means so much to me to know that I can always lean in and you'll be there, with your steady love and encouragement.

This book is for all of you who have been a part of the Vital Medicine community, especially the amazing individuals whom I have had the privilege to work with individually or in group. You have all been my teachers. Your unique journeys and embodied wisdom have guided me in cultivating the path and keys to vitality that I share here. Knowingly or not, we have been cartographers together in the creation of the Vitality Map.

A special thank you to all of the clients who gave me permission to share their stories in these pages—your stories are foundational to this book, and I'm deeply grateful! Through your vulnerability, authenticity, and courage, you are making possible the healing journeys of so many others.

And to my inaugural Vitality U cohort—you were the first clients to experience a deeply lived community of practice that reflected what I share here in *The Vitality Map*. Thank you for participating so fully and whole-heartedly. This experience not only catalyzed your own vitality journeys but also significantly nourished and encouraged me in my work. Words fall short of expressing my appreciation.

I am equally grateful to my Core Energetics community, who have held me so lovingly these last seven years—my fears, doubts, and vulnerabilities included—as I have grown into the woman capable of writing this book and bringing it into the world. You are family.

A special thank you to JoAnn Lovascio for the brilliant skill, grace, and embodied wisdom you have brought to my healing journey, truly helping me to find my voice and deeply align with my "yes" in life.

To Kristin and John for your incredible healing gifts. Thank you for guiding me to break through the patterns that were holding me back from expressing my light in the world.

To Dr. Nancy Welliver, a key player in my team of support. Your deep trust in my capacity to heal, through all the ups and downs of my journey, helped me to open into a long-term view of how to nourish my own vitality and cultivate my unique path.

To Dr. Brad Lichtenstein, a big thank you for your mentorship at Bastyr, for your support in my research for this book, and for all you have taught me and modeled for me.

To all the healthcare practitioners, teachers, mentors, and guides who have supported me on my learning and healing path. I've opened, developed, healed, and transformed with your guidance and support. You, too, are a part of the pages of this book, and I thank you.

To Ellen Daly, collaborative writer extraordinaire. Thank you for bringing your genius to this manuscript and helping to shape, refine, and finesse this book into its full beauty and potential. You have been like a book midwife for me. It has been such an honor and joy to work with you.

To Laura Didyk for navigating an iterative, cocreative copyediting journey with me, with patience, agility, and expert skill I could count on. Thank you for your grace and encouragement in the seemingly never-ending editing process. And to Sebastian Boensch for the fine-toothed comb you brought to my words, proofreading the manuscript with adept care and attention.

To Claudine Mansour for your incredible gift of design. You took my words and turned the outside and inside of *The Vitality Map* into a work of aesthetic beauty. Thank you for your gracious ability to compassionately stay with me in the cocreative process until I loved every aspect of the design.

To Joel Pitney for your amazing skills as a book-launch specialist. Your steady guidance, straight-up reflections, kindness, and encouragement were essential in navigating the myriad of decisions that needed to be made in order to connect my finished book with its audience. A deep bow of gratitude for your incredible presence through the labor and birth of this book.

To my first readers—Adam Ward, Lisa Brodsky, and Carlee Casey. I so deeply felt your love and care for me. You honored me and my work by giving of your time and energy in a vital and intimate way. Thank you for taking in what I shared so fully and for offering back your wisdom, honesty, and clear feedback, which helped to refine this book and give me greater confidence in letting others read it, too!

To all of the early endorsers of this book. Baron Short, Terry Patten, Lynne Feldman, Karen Wyatt, Georgia Tetlow, Rob McNamara, Maureen Metcalf, Vicki Robin, and Michael Finkelstein, your overwhelming enthusiasm and encouragement and your grace-filled words helped me move through the vulnerability of bringing this book into the world, while also inspiring me to reach out for further support and endorsements.

To all of my dear friends and family who opened their homes to me during the nomadic time that was a part of the creative flow in writing this book. Leslie and George Johnson, Christina and Ben Greené, Gayle Livingston and Steven LaCroix, Aimee Huyck and Adam Myers, Lisa Brodsky, Kippy Messett, Dana Carman, Miriam and Stephan Martineau, and, of course, Sharon and Elliot Zucker, your love and generosity are alive in the pages of this book.

To Abigail Lynam for witnessing and loving me like a sister through so many teary and vulnerable conversations, celebrations, and transitions. You have been such a dear friend and support in my life.

To Adam Ward for being an intimate part of the writing and emergence of this book. Thank you for your consistent support and encouragement, for all of your reflections and input, and, most importantly, for your sincere, unfaltering, loving belief in me. I'm grateful for your presence in my life, your kindness, and your generosity of spirit.

And to all of my dear friends, near and far, new and old, too many to name and honor as I'd like. I feel so deeply blessed by every one of you. You each have held, influenced, challenged, opened, witnessed, embraced, loved, and nurtured me in my growth, healing, and ongoing evolution. You each have helped to shape the woman I am, and thus the words on these pages. Thank you.

FOREWORD

For many years, as I rose through the ranks of the medical profession and built my career as a successful doctor, I was haunted by the feeling that something was missing. Although my patients thanked me and my peers honored my work, I felt out of place in my own medical practice and the systems in which I worked. I came to realize that I wasn't really healing people. I was just giving them quick fixes, in the form of pills, prescriptions, and procedures, and sooner or later, they would come back for more. The principle reason for this revolving door was that I, like most doctors, was not really teaching people how to live healthy lives. So I ventured beyond the medical establishment and launched a personal quest to become a true healer and a true teacher, giving people the tools they need to live skillfully.

I am happy to have met a kindred spirit in Deborah Zucker—someone who brings wisdom and thoughtfulness to the complex riddle of human health. The title of this book promises something we all long for: Vitality. And yet as much as that word may evoke feelings of energy, dynamism, and vigor, Deborah understands an important truth: that sometimes, to get well means to slow down.

In this age of too much information, we are subjected to a nonstop barrage of stress-inducing images and messages. In addition, with everything moving at lightning speed, we are under constant strain to perform and produce around the clock. For these reasons, many of us hit fight-or-flight mode shortly after opening our eyes and keep at it until we collapse into bed at night. Some of us never even exit this state and are therefore unable to sleep well, despite how exhausted we feel.

Our state of exhaustion on the macro level is a reflection of what is going on at the micro, or cellular, level. Our sympathetic nervous system is wired to handle some stress, but not to be locked in the "on" position, the way it is in our modern world. As a result of our go-go-go lifestyles today, our natural reserves of vitamins, minerals, and enzymes—all of which we need to stay energized and healthy—are getting depleted.

This becomes quite evident when our bodies succumb to illness, and when our minds are preoccupied with troubling thoughts and feelings of

anxiety and dis-ease. The medical establishment, presumptively here to re-
lieve us from these states, is unable to handle all of it, leaving many, if not
most, in distress. Increasingly, many turn to alternatives, but they too, especially those emphasizing simplistic "remedies," let us down.

The fact is that in order to find genuine relief, there is a bigger picture
that requires our attention. And neither the body nor the mind need to be
in perfect shape to achieve this. Instead, what we need is an approach to
living that addresses the whole of it, including the pain, the suffering, and
the death. This is humbling to consider. It may even feel like a form of surrender to these great forces that affect and limit our lifespan. But, they do
not have to ruin our lives.

The fact is, you are not your disease, or your mortal condition, no matter how you define it. The you inside, the witness observing what is taking place, is a deep-seated consciousness that will transcend the problems.
What you need is not a quick fix, then, but rather a slow and conscientious
process of engagement in the one life you have, allowing you to live it to
the fullest. And for that, you need wisdom, which is what you will find in
these pages.

Deborah Zucker has pulled together the science of life and a highly intelligent and comprehensive understanding of living. She understands that
we all need something practical to hold onto, especially as we venture away
from the crowd (which happens to be heading off a cliff in its desperation
for short-term solutions). With both courage and integrity she offers a sustainable way to move in the other direction. She offers a map for a relationship with life that helps us deal with our challenges—not only through
relieving some of the associated suffering but through allowing us to immediately sense the beauty as it unfolds around us in our hope-filled journey
back to wholeness.

What I like about Deborah's writing is the honest voice of a caring practitioner who presents herself as a fellow traveler more than an authority. It
is the latter that, for me, gives her the greatest credibility, though her formal
training in the healing arts also goes a long way toward assuring the reader
they are in good hands. She freely shares her own insight and knowledge,
but she also does something more important: she connects readers with
their own deeper intelligence and the wisdom of the body. With her personal and professional experience, she guides us to check in to the body-mind
source of our awareness—to feel more completely and to transform any

anxiety into action that makes sense.

Along the way, she invites us to reflect on questions of personal inquiry; key among them is, "What brings you vitally alive," a question that emphasizes the inner wisdom, unique purpose, and passions we each possess. And she urges us to remain playful and curious despite the seriousness of the project, leading us away from the tendency to be too harsh a critic of our own progress. Instead, she compassionately counsels us to experiment, to learn, and to see this as a process—one that is insightful and thoughtful as well as practical.

I agree with Deborah—there are several keys to success, and I like how she frames the work in that way. Her book is digestible, and while the path is not entirely easy, it is actually simple enough. I think you will find this book a refreshing alternative to many of the simplistic "how-to" books so common these days. We human beings are wiser than we may realize. While we may instinctively look for quick relief, we know that shortcuts and Band-Aids don't work. Our bodies and our innate intelligence will appreciate the deep truth of the plan that Deborah lays out in *The Vitality Map*.

—MICHAEL B. FINKELSTEIN, M.D.,
author of *Slow Medicine*

Every part of you is welcome here
From cells to bones to spirit
From everyday challenges to ancient wisdom
Your stories, beliefs, hopes, dreams, and fears
Your community, your solitude,
and your sacred relationship with yourself

INTRODUCTION

I COULDN'T STOP CRYING. Lying in my bed in the fetal position, I could hear my friends joking around as they cooked dinner downstairs. I felt exhausted, awful, and their happy voices just made me feel worse. I was twenty-four years old, living in a community of wonderful people who shared my passions and my values, and yet, for no reason that I could name, my life felt like it was spinning out of control.

A few weeks earlier, seemingly without warning, I had spiraled rapidly into deep fatigue and depression. I'd had blood tests done, gone to see a series of conventional doctors, and had consultations with alternative practitioners—I was swimming in the confusion of it all. The diagnoses they'd given me didn't seem to explain the depth of my fatigue and my relatively sudden emotional dive.

In that moment, as I lay in my bed in this home I loved, I came to the realization that I was going to have to stay with my parents for awhile. I needed a different kind of space to figure out what this health crisis was about for me, I needed to rest, recover, and find my way to healing so I could move forward. I felt the truth of that need, and then felt the requisite shame that came with it. How could I—the energetic, enthusiastic, world-changing overachiever—be in this situation? I should be in my prime. I should be able to rally. And yet I couldn't even get out of bed.

For months, much of that time living with my parents, I was so tired that just walking around the block each day was a huge feat. Ironically, the community where I was living and working when this began was a sustainability education center in Oregon. I was helping to heal our world, yet hadn't learned how to treat myself with the same care. Sure, I was eating organic, growing my own food, exercising daily, living among supportive friends, doing work that felt important, and yet, surprisingly, these things weren't enough.

In retrospect, I can clearly see all the warning signs that had been there for months, even years. I can now see the level of stress I was living under, much of which was created by my high expectations for myself. Because I hadn't learned how to acknowledge, feel, and share the full range of my emotions and reactions, I was tightly wound and contained, using so much energy to maintain a particular persona. Vulnerability was my greatest fear. I didn't know how to let others in, to ask for support, to cry and be held, to acknowledge my fears and anxiety, or to express anger.

What began as chronic fatigue, depression, and a host of other ailments quickly evolved into an intimate encounter with every level of my being: body, psyche, emotions, and spirit. The experience, uncomfortable as it was, also became an eye-opening and educational tour through the spectrum of both ancient and modern healing modalities. Becoming a doctor had never been part of my plan, but the healer in me had awakened, and there was no putting it back to sleep. Even when I could barely get out of bed, I felt compelled to share what I was learning about health and healing with others. I felt truly called to guide others through their often lonely and scary healing transitions.

Thus began my Naturopathic medical training at Bastyr University and my own spiritual quest to create a path to health and vitality that takes into account the wholeness and uniqueness of each individual, while being deeply rooted in nature and community—two foundational pillars of my own experience of healing holistically. While I found ways to adapt and function at a fairly "normal" level during my doctorate training, my personal health challenges continued and were intimately woven into my medical studies. It took many years of being chronically ill, repeating unconscious patterns in relation to my own self-care, even relapsing into a period of deep fatigue after I was a licensed physician, to awaken to and refine my own healing navigation tool—the Vitality Map—which I will share with you in this book.

My own health journey, with all its ups and downs, is at the core of my approach to healing. I consider myself a "wounded healer," meaning that I bring forth everything I've learned and become on my journey to support and empower you on yours. I am intimate with the landscape and its obstacles, and what it takes to move across it and through life with more ease and aliveness. I know how important it is to feel greater alignment and wholeness, and how essential it is to increase your capacity to nourish and empower yourself along your healing journey.

Today, I feel more vital and at home in myself than ever before. I hold a soft, compassionate space for the entire range of this human experience— the light *and* the dark. I understand transitions, challenges, and topsy-turvy times—and I know they hold within them the possibility for great awakenings, renewed vitality, and deeper connections.

I believe "health" is the sum of your entire experience in this life. It's not just the number you see when you stand on the scale, the lunch you had yesterday, or whether you can successfully do a downward dog pose in your yoga class. It's everything—from your intimate relationships to your spiritual practice to how you talk to yourself when no one's listening. It all matters—every single part of you and your unique, precious life.

My main mission—the thing that lights me up most—is helping conscious, compassionate people revolutionize their health by learning how to love, nourish, and heal themselves, on every level, so they can show up fully to help heal our world.

Through my Vital Medicine work, I mentor individuals and groups in many virtual and retreat-based programs, including private Skype mentoring, an intimate nine-month small-cohort program, wilderness mini vision quests, online home-study courses, and continuing-education programs for health practitioners. I am grateful through these pages to now have the opportunity and the platform to share what I've learned with readers like you who long for greater vitality.

In this book you will receive guidance and encouragement in how to:

✦ Stop beating yourself up over all the things you think you "should" be doing to get healthy, and instead learn to listen to what your body truly needs.

✦ Peacefully conquer your self-sabotaging habits, and make sustainable changes to create the life you're meant to live.

✦ Move into a more vibrant relationship with yourself and the web of relationships that support you.

✦ Stop trying to fix yourself, and step into an entirely new, positive, and deeply reverent relationship with your own self-care.

✦ Let go of what no longer belongs in your life and experience the freedom and ease to focus on what truly brings you alive.

◆ Experience a profound shift into a new relationship with yourself, your body, and your life journey—a shift marked by deep integration, wholeness, and nurturing self-care.

I am not promising you a quick fix, and I have no interest in sharing a prescription that might help for a few weeks until the realities of your daily life kick in, and this journey becomes yet another thing to add to your growing list of shame-building internal failures. This is a guidebook for the long haul, for help in reaching, practicing, and experiencing *sustainable* health and vitality.

These days, we're overwhelmed with a deluge of theories and tips that claim to be the keys to health, and we can spend years, if not decades, bouncing between the latest fads—diets, exercise programs, supplements, therapies, and on and on. But until we address what is going on *at the foundational level of our relationship with health and how we care for ourselves*, we will forever be disconnected from our potential to truly thrive and flourish.

The 9 Keys to Deep Vitality are meant to support you in revolutionizing your health and life, *starting at the foundation*. This book will guide you to drop into a deeper, more authentic relationship with yourself, and with life itself. By investing in creating a strong foundation you invest in changing your whole approach to life, in how you make everyday choices regarding your self-care, your work, and your relationships. It will transform your priorities. Living with the guidance of these keys offers you the opportunity to feel empowered in skillfully caring for yourself and aligning your life at a level that you may have never known.

Throughout this book, I share stories from real people I've worked with that demonstrate the kind of transformation that is possible when you embrace your self-care and compassion at the deepest levels. While names and details have been changed to protect identities, the problems these people have faced and the shifts they've experienced are absolutely authentic. I hope that seeing how they were able to turn their lives and their health around will inspire you to realize that you can do the same.

Why waste another day, another hour, another second feeling trapped or unhappy in your body, in your life? You can accomplish deep, radically positive shifts with less effort and fewer tears than you think. It simply takes willingness, commitment, and deep support. I'd be honored to support you, wherever you are in your life's journey.

HOW TO USE THIS BOOK

Before I head out on any extended backcountry wilderness journey I always take time to study the map and get a feel for the territory I'm heading into. Doing so gives me a sense of how to pace myself, what to bring along, and where I plan to camp each night. Even if things change along the way, I feel safer and more relaxed when I have the sense that I know how to confidently guide myself to where I want to go. In the same way, this Vitality Map can help you to see the big picture and topography of your unique health journey.

Please take your time as you move through these pages. The Vitality Map offers the opportunity for a significant restructuring of your internal navigation system, and it's a process that needs time and space to unfold. The 9 Keys to Deep Vitality open the doors into the territory of the Vitality Map and serve as a framework for you to follow. Each key builds upon the next, and they are meant to be read in order, at least initially. Once you are familiar with them, I think you'll find you'll want to return to individual keys, depending on where you are on your health journey and with the larger process and flow of the entire Vitality Map, to dive even deeper into their wisdom.

Each key has its own chapter, and I'd suggest giving yourself the spaciousness to read no more than one key a week to allow time to integrate, steep, and let the words penetrate deeper into the realities of your day-to-day life.

As I've said, this guide is about the long haul. There's no hurry. I encourage you to trust your own self-knowing in this. You might integrate the material better if you read it through once initially at a steady pace to get an overview of the territory, then return to explore the material more intimately and with spaciousness to incorporate the learning into your daily life. Only you can know for yourself what you need, and what will best support your transformative process. You are your own best guide, and if there is one thing I hope you will take away from this book, it is greater confidence in that fact.

The Vitality Map offers you the chance to experience a truly transformative journey—one that will help you reclaim your energy, joy, and vitality and begin to live in your fullest natural expression. I've designed the book to support you in engaging intimately and experientially with the material I present, not to remain in an intellectual, detached stance. I will give you ample opportunity to practice, experiment, and inquire.

If you'd like, take a moment now to settle in and allow yourself to arrive in the calm and safety of this space. Perhaps you can close your eyes and take a few conscious breaths. Let yourself feel what's present for you right now.

What is it that you are yearning for? What is it that you hope this book may offer you in your life? Are you longing to feel more vital? Are you overwhelmed, exhausted, too busy to take care of yourself in the ways you'd like to? Are you feeling as if you've tried everything—pills, detoxes, diets—to bring more energy, ease, and strength into your life, but nothing seems to work?

If so, please know that you're not alone. Almost everyone who comes to work with me feels similarly. And as I've shared already, I know intimately how frustrating it is to not feel good in your body or to feel out of alignment in your life—and I've learned through my own healing journey how to change it.

Your journey will be unique and particular to you, and there is no book that can predict every twist and turn of your path. As the old saying goes, the map is not the territory. But maps can be tremendously useful in orienting us to the general contours of the landscape. When we discover a map of somewhere we have never been, it can be like opening a door to a whole new world.

CHECKING IN

Each of the chapters will include a "check-in," a suggestion to take a moment and be present with yourself in the midst of your reading. This will be an opportunity to pause in the consumption of the material and inquire within, becoming more aware of and intimate with the reactions, openings, and insights that may be arising. Think of the check-ins as little nudges to drop deeper into yourself and integrate and embody what you are reading. The check-ins offer you an opportunity to strengthen your awareness muscles. I hope this practice will be something you carry into your daily life, making you more conscious of your reactions and insights, shifts and changes that might be happening, and the feedback that your body is giving you all the time.

OPPORTUNITIES FOR ENGAGEMENT

Woven throughout all of the chapters are inquiry questions, meditations, guided visualizations, and suggested practices designed to help you engage with the ideas in a direct, intimate, and personal way. I want to provide you with as many opportunities as possible to enter into a process that is alive, dynamic, transformative, and healing. Much can happen simply by encountering the ideas in each chapter and letting them percolate in your consciousness. Yet if you feel ready to begin applying them concretely, I have no doubt that you will find yourself coming alive in ways you never expected.

TOOLS TO SUPPORT YOU ON YOUR JOURNEY

JOURNAL: Throughout the book, I will guide you through inquiry processes. I'd recommend buying a special journal that is dedicated solely to your exploration here.

VITALITY BUDDY: Later in the book we'll discuss the importance of having support on your journey. A simple way to start receiving support now is to reach out to your friends and see who might be interested in going through *The Vitality Map* and the exercises with you. You might even introduce them to the possibility by gifting them a copy of the book.

VITALITY DATES: I'd encourage you to create dedicated time each week—to make a date with yourself (or with your Vitality Buddy)—for devoting yourself to the practices offered in each chapter. Schedule it into your calendar and head to an inspiring spot in nature, a quiet place in your home, or your favorite coffee shop.

PERSONAL & PROFESSIONAL SUPPORT: Along the way, you may find that in order to move forward with this journey, you may need or want to reach out for different kinds of support. Pay attention to your inner guidance as you are reading and make sure that you ask for the support you need, whether it be professional help or encouragement from your loved ones.

ADDITIONAL RESOURCES

To accompany this book, I've created a multimedia package that includes free resources to support and deepen your experiential healing journey. You'll find:

- ✦ A PDF workbook (which you can print and write in, or work with on your computer) with the inquiry questions from each chapter

- ✦ Audio recordings of the meditations

- ✦ PDF summaries of the 9 Keys to Deep Vitality (ready to be printed out as reminders)

- ✦ Spreadsheets to use for awareness practices

- ✦ And more . . .

Go to **www.thevitalitymap.com/gift** (or scan the QR code below) to gain access to these gifts, and look for the following symbols throughout the book to indicate when these additional resources on specific topics are available to you:

 indicates that there is an audio recording available to download.

 indicates that you can find the written exercise in the PDF workbook.

CHAPTER 1

WHAT'S BECOME OF YOUR VITALITY?

"Unbeing dead isn't being alive."
—E.E. CUMMINGS

THE VOICE ON the other end of the phone sounded close to breaking. "I'm feeling completely exhausted. I have to drag myself to work each day. And not only that, but the depression I had in my twenties has returned in full force this fall." I could hear that the tears had started to flow. "It all feels so messed up."

The voice and the tears belonged to Amy, a longtime friend of mine. It had been about ten years since we had been in touch, but she'd recently reached out to me for support. She sounded desperate.

Amy is forty-five years old, married, with two children ages five and ten, and lives in Portland, Oregon, where she has her own business as a life coach.

"I'm so sorry to hear you're having such a rough time," I told her. "From what I could see on your Facebook posts, everything seemed to be going great."

"That's just the thing—it is!" she responded. "My kids are amazing, and I feel so blessed to be a mom. My business is doing great—my clientele comes almost entirely from referrals at this point. And I love my husband and the home we've created together. I spend my days supporting others in making choices to create lives they love, and I pour out all of this energy to nurture my kids as they blossom into the unique people that they are, but I feel completely lost. I feel like I should know by now how to find my way back and that I shouldn't be feeling like I do. Who am I to be miserable and depressed when I have so much to be grateful for? It's crazy, right?"

Amy's story didn't sound crazy to me at all. It was heart-wrenching and, sadly, very familiar. I hear so many stories just like Amy's, from clients, friends, and loved ones—so much so that it feels like an epidemic is happening. On the outside, things look great—a beautiful family, a loving relationship, a fulfilling career of serving and helping others. And yet at a deeper, more foundational level there is something missing—something that would allow Amy, or any of us, to feel alive, vital, and thriving. I can say from my personal and professional experience that that elusive something is directly connected to how we care for ourselves.

If I were to boil it down to one word, I would choose "vitality." We all have within us an innate life-energy that infuses us, a force within that naturally wishes us to express, grow, move, heal, and evolve. And yet, in the same way that the energy of a wild animal diminishes when it is put into a cage at the zoo, our own vitality may not have the conditions, nourishment, and freedom it needs in order to fully express itself in our lives.

The details of the story are different for each of us—what specific issues we find ourselves struggling with—and yet there are similar patterns I've seen in our underlying relationship with our own self-care. In the midst of all the modern advances in medicine, it seems that so many of us live with a baffling sense of *dis*-ease, a knowing that we are not experiencing the level of health and well-being that we know is possible.

I'm certainly not the only one to notice this epidemic of vitality loss. In the business world, it's called, aptly, "burnout." A Harvard Medical School study found that an astonishing 96 percent of leaders felt burned out.[1] Arianna Huffington, who charts this phenomenon in great detail in her book *Thrive,* offers a host of statistics showing how widespread burnout is, and the impacts it has on our happiness, health, and well-being. For example, she points out that in the United Kingdom prescriptions for antidepressants have gone up 495 percent since 1991.[2] She goes on to share that US employers are shelling out 200 to 300 percent more on healthcare related to reduced productivity, sick days, and absenteeism than they are on direct healthcare costs.[3] And in Germany the labor minister estimated that they were losing ten billion euros per year on burnout. Reflecting on all of this research, Arianna concludes, "Burnout, stress, and depression have become worldwide epidemics."[4]

Does any of this sound familiar to you? Perhaps you're not taking antidepressants, or getting out of bed is not a problem for you, but I wonder if you've recently uttered any of these phrases that I hear all the time from clients and loved ones:

"I'm too busy to . . . "

"I feel like I should know better."

"I am embarrassed to admit . . . "

"I'm lazy. I can't seem to keep any new healthy habit going."

"I've tried everything—pills, diets, exercise routines—and nothing really works."

"I'm so confused about what to do to take care of myself. I feel spun around with all the conflicting information out there. Each week there's something new to do."

"I feel lost and out of control."

"I don't know who I am anymore."

"I want to feel energized and alive, yet I don't know how to get there from here."

"I'm tired of the boom and bust cycle in how I care for myself."

"I feel like true health is always out of reach."

"I used to feel energized and unstoppable, but it has been a long time since I felt that way."

I have a feeling that for every person who I hear say these things, there are so many more who have these kinds of thoughts, self-judgments, and shame about how they are or aren't caring for themselves and yet have not shared those sentiments with anyone.

I have the honor of working with many smart, compassionate, capable people. These are folks who are out there doing so much good in the world—leading organizations, supporting others as healers and teachers, activists and consultants, mothers and fathers. Outwardly, these people may look like they have it all together, yet I get to hear the inner stories: how they have felt embarrassed and struggled for years with their weight; how they've been hooked on sleep medication for too long because they are riddled with anxiety in the night; how they have had a secret addiction to cigarettes for the last twenty-five years; how they feel ashamed that they can't seem to get over their resistance to exercise; how they haven't had sex with their spouse for years. It seems that no one is immune to these secret sources of shame, no matter how evolved or competent they may seem.

What I have observed is that other than sharing these secrets with a health practitioner like myself (in the way of a confessional), most of us rarely, if ever, say out loud to another person the vulnerable truth of what is really going on for us in our relationship with self-care—the frustration, the confusion, the embarrassment, and the shame. Even if we occasionally confide in a professional, there is a sense of isolation, a compartmentalization where we don't open up to our friends and loved ones about our struggles. The irony is that if we did, we'd probably discover that we are not alone at all. Most of us, in our own way, are struggling to achieve and sustain the changes we need in order to feel more alive and vital.

The cost of the isolation and the shame is huge. We can find ourselves in a self-perpetuating cycle as we become trapped in our self-judgments and pain about our inability to create and sustain change—the loud voices within reinforce the behavior patterns and then the behavior patterns reinforce the loud voices. When it comes to our perceived failures in the realm of self-care, we rarely take the risk to be vulnerable and, because of this, we unwittingly keep ourselves locked in unhealthy patterns.

One of the most insightful writers on the topic of shame and vulnerability is Brené Brown, and I have come to lean on her wisdom often in my work with clients because she cuts right to the heart of what is going on for so many of us. I particularly appreciate how she normalizes shame. She writes, "People often want to believe that shame is reserved for people who have survived an unspeakable trauma, but this is not true. Shame is something we all experience."[5] She goes on to share the twelve shame categories that she has identified in her research. The top shame inducer for women is appearance and body image. Others inducers include mental and physical health, addiction, sex, and aging.[6]

I see all of these sources of shame among my clients, both women and men. Brown has also researched and written extensively on the topic of vulnerability, and how it is our greatest fear and the thing that will help us heal:

> Our rejection of vulnerability often stems from our associating it with dark emotions like fear, shame, grief, sadness, and disappointment, emotions we don't want to discuss. . . . What most of us fail to understand, and what took me a decade of research to learn is that vulnerability is also the cradle of the emotions and experiences we crave. Vulnerability is the birthplace of love, belonging, joy, courage, empathy, and creativity. It is the source of hope, empathy, accountability, and authenticity.[7]

Brown points out that vulnerability about our weaknesses is key to actually changing the very things we're ashamed of, including our health challenges. "From the field of health psychology," she writes, "studies show that perceived vulnerability, meaning the ability to acknowledge our risks and exposure, greatly increases our chances of adhering to some kind of positive health regimen. In order to get patients to comply with prevention routines, they must work on perceived vulnerability."[8]

If you're struggling with the kinds of issues I've been describing in this chapter—if, like my friend Amy, you feel exhausted, depressed, and desperate, but ashamed of yourself for feeling that way—I hope that what I am sharing here serves as an invitation to you to be vulnerable, even if only with yourself. Our lack of vulnerability tends to start with ourselves, with the perceived failings we are ashamed to admit even in the privacy of our own minds. Now is the time to be gentle with yourself, to stop beating yourself up inwardly about all those things you know you "should" be doing, or all the things you think you "shouldn't" be feeling.

CHECKING IN: *Pause for a moment to check in. How are you feeling physically in this moment? Emotionally? What is being evoked for you by what you have been reading so far?*

THE BODHISATTVA SYNDROME

Once Amy let herself admit to me how desperate she was feeling, and how ashamed she was of feeling that way, I started asking questions to find out more about what was going on. The picture that emerged is a common one. Amy had been juggling being a mom with starting and running her business for the last nine years. While her husband is a very nurturing man, she felt that when the kids came into the picture, he channeled that nurturing energy to them. They parented well together, yet she felt a distance with him, a lack of the intimacy that she yearned for. And while she could see that her clients were benefiting from working with her, she felt disconnected from her passion in her work. It was like the fire had gone out.

"It all feels like too much," she told me. "I am always running from this thing to that, juggling everything. I feel overwhelmed, like there is never enough time. I know all of the things I should do to take care of myself that will probably make me feel better, yet I never can seem to get around to them or sustain the changes if I do try something. My exercise is sporadic at best. I know that I have been leaning on food to try to make me feel better, and I have been gaining weight for a while now. My sleep no longer feels refreshing. I wake up tired. My digestion seems to be all messed up. I feel like I'm falling apart. I'm so frightened and anxious that things will continue to spiral down, and feel more out of control and out of balance and then I won't be able to find my way back up. I don't know how to make it all stop. My doctor wants to put me on an antidepressant, but that doesn't feel like the answer."

As she spoke, it was clear to me that Amy didn't need drugs—she just needed the kind of support and nurturing that she was constantly giving to others. I suggested this to her, and there was a long silence in which I heard her struggling to stem the flow of tears. Finally, she said, "You, know, you're right. It feels kind of selfish, but recently I've found myself thinking, 'What about me?'"

Amy's predicament reflects a pattern that I see so often (and have certainly known in myself), in which it can be so much easier to care for others than to care for ourselves, to support everyone around us than to reach out for support for ourselves. I've playfully come to call this the Bodhisattva Syndrome.

In the Buddhist tradition, a Bodhisattva is someone who gives his or her life to compassionate service to reduce the suffering of all sentient beings. The term Bodhisattva Syndrome is my way to point to how, in our earnest desire to serve and benefit others, we often sacrifice ourselves in ways that are counterproductive to our intentions. Self-sacrifice and martyrdom are well reinforced culturally even amongst the most conscious and self-aware leaders and teachers.

It honestly breaks my heart to see how entrenched these beliefs and behavior patterns can be. When I reflected to Amy that it sounded like she needed to be held, too, she agreed, but with tentativeness, as if it were uncomfortable for her to acknowledge this and say it out loud. She had been having thoughts along these lines but had told herself she was just being selfish.

I've noticed that women, with our hardwired propensity to nurture, are more likely to fall prey to the Bodhisattva Syndrome, especially those who are juggling a family and a career. But I've seen the same symptoms in plenty of men as well. Last summer I met Daniel, a man in his late forties who was just getting back on his feet after devoting a decade of his life to caring for two disabled parents, putting his own life's dreams on hold. The self-sacrifice culminated in extreme sleep deprivation while doing nighttime care for his mother during an extended fourteen-month hospice journey. It took him two years to emerge from the fatigue that enveloped him.

What I wish for is that we can become the Bodhisattvas who do not forsake ourselves. We can include our own welfare in our service—whether it be as parents, in our work, how we show up with friends, or the ways in which we volunteer in our communities. If we exclude ourselves from our own circle of care, we shortchange not only our own health and well-being, but also those we want to care for most. Amy, like so many people I know, was finding herself spiraling down and away from her own sense of thriving with such momentum that it felt impossible to reverse. There's nothing sustainable about this, nor does it benefit her kids, loved ones, clients, or community. How valuable and helpful are her gifts if she runs herself into the ground trying to offer them?

PERSONAL SUSTAINABILITY

What I shared with Amy that day is the idea of personal sustainability. In a culture that reinforces the ideal of self-sacrifice, we often prioritize caring for others and caring for our world, while we view caring for ourselves as being somehow in opposition to that ideal, even interpreting it as being selfish or narcissistic. And yet what I'm talking about here has nothing to do with narcissism or selfishness. In fact, the sentiment is quite the opposite. Personal sustainability is about caring for ourselves in such a way that we have more to give and more energy to serve.

Personal sustainability means to me that we hold a long-term perspective on our lives. Our self-care is about the long haul, and over time, self-sacrifice serves no one. Running ourselves into the ground is a losing strategy both for ourselves and for the people we care about. We can only serve and care for others if we have consciously cultivated our own foundation of health.

From this perspective, self-care and care for others are not opposite poles, but inextricably linked. We live our days replenishing and renewing ourselves through how we care for ourselves so that we can continue to show up in service to others and our world. For me, this becomes an authentic and holistic Bodhisattva vow where we recognize that we are in service to life, and that each human being (including ourselves) is part of life; we each matter.

Whether you are just beginning to recognize these symptoms and patterns at play or are already way down the rabbit hole like Amy, I'm glad you found your way here. I wrote this book, and the keys in it, to meet you wherever you are and help you to create a new foundation of empowered self-care that gives you the roots and capacity to show up in the world to support and serve the needs of yourself and others, as well as our collective future.

SEEING WITH CLEAR EYES

If you are like Amy and my other clients, you probably already have a pretty clear idea of what your individual struggles are in relation to your health and the quality of your self-care. You may not have ever voiced them, but deep down you know what they are. My hope is that with a little bit of guidance and support from the Vitality Map to bring things to the surface, you will become more aware of what deeply nourishes you and brings you alive—what feeds your sense of vitality. Some of this awareness may be front and center in your mind—you see it and feel it every single day (and it might not be comfortable)—while some of it may be just beneath the surface, showing up every so often. Other parts of it may be things that you've known and acknowledged to yourself but haven't consciously thought about for years.

As we begin this journey together, I invite you to take a moment to begin to see with clear eyes where you are now, acknowledging those elements that are right on the surface as well as those that are a little buried. I know from my own healing and learning experiences that it is difficult to dive into new waters, to fully open myself to the growth opportunities available to me, if I haven't first come into a direct, clear, authentic relationship with the waters I'm currently swimming in.

INQUIRY QUESTIONS

I invite you now to grab your journal and give yourself the gift of 30 minutes to explore the following questions:

+ What does the word "vitality" mean to you?

+ What are your passions? What do you love to do? What makes you come alive?

+ If you were to imagine nourishing and unleashing your innate vitality, what would that look/feel like to you? Write a list of activities that you know nourish your vitality. If you can't think of any, try to remember the last time you felt yourself come alive: What were you doing? Who were you with? Describe the scene.

+ In this moment, if you were to create a list of things that stifle your vitality, what would you include?

+ How does your daily life reflect these two lists? Is it weighted more on one side or the other? And what changes might you need to make in order to unleash your vitality?

+ What potential obstacles do you foresee in implementing the life changes you seek?

+ Who do you know who could sincerely and consistently support you as you embark on this transformative healing path?

CHAPTER 2

RETURNING TO WHOLENESS

❖

*"When we have the awareness that we are not what we think—
this is the first step to recovering what we truly are."*
—DON MIGUEL RUIZ

WHILE ON A HIKE with my friend Joel, a newly licensed physician who had recently started his first medical practice, he confessed to me, as we walked along a beautiful forest trail, that he was feeling some disillusionment about his chosen profession and generally feeling lost in life.

"I always dreamed of being a doctor. I've spent the past four years working my ass off in med school to get here," he said wryly, "and now look at me. I'm wondering what I've gotten myself into. Whatever we call the 'healthcare' system just doesn't feel meaningful to me. I barely get to spend any time with my patients. I can tell there are deeper issues going on with many of them that I just don't have the capacity or permission to address. And I find myself falling back on 'quick-fix' solutions that I know aren't really getting to the root of the problem. I feel like there's so much more to health than what I'm allowed to practice in my clinic."

Although the healthcare profession is filled with wonderful, caring, dedicated professionals like Joel, the system itself has significant limitations. And at the heart of those limitations is the way the system defines health. In this chapter we'll explore and expand our definition of health beyond the narrow confines of physical symptomology.

But first, let me ask you: When you think about *health* what are the first things that come to mind? In your journal, write down the words that arise, or if you don't feel like writing now, simply pause for a minute and listen to the words that come up. The key is to not censor yourself, so you can see what beliefs and associations you have that might not be in your conscious awareness.

When I ask this question in workshops that I teach, some of the common responses are:

"Going to the gym."

"Eating salads every day."

"Being able to sleep through the night."

"Not getting sick all the time."

"Living pain-free."

"Going to see my doctor."

"Having enough energy to do the things I want to do."

When I look at these answers, they fall into two categories: 1) things people believe they "should" be doing in order to be healthy, and 2) experiences and states of being connected to their physical bodies.

Many people relate to their health with a kind of managerial energy—managing and taking care of their physical bodies so that they feel good and do not get sick. When they fall short of the unreasonably high expectations this approach tends to cultivate, they feel inadequate and ashamed.

In this approach, health becomes one more practical aspect of our lives to attend to—right alongside things like cleaning our houses, doing the laundry, driving the kids to school, going to work, and studying for our exams.

A standard definition of health is simply being free from disease or physical pain. Granted, many practitioners will expand that definition to include emotional, psychological, and even spiritual pain, but when you show up at your doctor's office, the odds are that he or she is going to be focused primarily on the physical symptoms. And you probably are too. When you take the kind of "managerial" approach I described above, you go to a doctor with the same kind of orientation with which you'd go to a car mechanic—to get a tune-up, or to find out what's wrong. Obviously, you are not a car. You are not mechanistic and cannot be reduced down to your organs, blood, hormones, neurochemicals, skin, and bones. This expression of life that is you is so much more than that.

A more helpful and accurate approach to health includes all of who you are, putting health at the foundation and center of your life and your life-force. Health, to me, is about what brings you vitally alive, helps you connect with your truth and with your authentic self. No part of your lived existence can be isolated from the other parts—every aspect of your physical body, the activities you engage in every day, how you feel and respond to others and the world, who you relate to and how you connect, and what makes you uniquely you—all of these are woven together into one beautiful, complex whole: YOU!

While we delineate all the different aspects of who we are, using labels like "mind," "body," "soul," "emotions," and "spirit," even the language itself creates boundaries where there are none. Those words can be helpful in some circumstances, yet YOU are one whole, and those parts of you that we talk about can't be explored, examined, observed, and "diagnosed" as separate entities.

So if you relate to health as simply managing your physical body through eating broccoli, going to yoga class, running three miles a day, and showing up for your annual physical, it is only going to lead you to unending frustration. Sure, those things can contribute to your state of vitality, but so does every single choice you make, every day of your life. If you think that managing your physical body in these ways is all you need to be doing for your health, you'll be in an endless chase, searching for the next thing you need to do to increase your vitality, and completely missing the bigger, more extraordinary reality you are part of.

Separating out our mental and emotional states, our spiritual paths, our intimate relationships, or our work in the world from our "health" draws false distinctions that create fragmentation where there is none. Your relationship to health is inextricably linked to your relationship with every aspect of your life. If you are struggling in work, it is going to affect your state of vitality. If you are navigating a relationship transition, it is going to affect your state of vitality. Health is every aspect of you and your unique life—how you live, breathe, work, relate, and serve.

COMING HOME TO THE WHOLE OF WHO YOU ARE

The true definition of health does not mean merely "without pathology." It is not simply the absence of pain or disease. In fact, I believe it actually necessitates that we embrace our mortality, diseases, aging, and emotional and physical ups and downs as part of our health journey. We live in a culture that boils down our symptoms into pathology, disease, and diagnoses. Yet it is possible, and more productive and helpful, to view symptoms as feedback, signals of a realignment that is wanting to happen. We can view our *dis*-ease as part of the generative life wisdom within us. If you're accustomed to looking at health in a narrower way, this may feel like a huge paradigm shift, yet it's one that I trust will be life-giving.

In fact, this is not a "new" definition of health at all—quite the opposite. Did you know that the Germanic word root for "health" actually means "whole"? Michael Finkelstein, MD, offers a beautiful definition of health that encompasses this original meaning in his book *Slow Medicine*: "Health is a natural state of wholeness, marked by the establishment of a dynamic balance, encompassing and fully integrating the areas of our mental/emotional, physical, spiritual, social, and environmental condition."[9]

In line with this understanding, my approach to health is about coming home to the whole of who you are. Health is the ground of life, the foundation underlying everything. Health is about cultivating the soil of your life, the soil that allows your natural, innate life-energy to guide you to blossom and bloom in the world.

WHAT IS SELF-CARE AND WHY IS IT SUCH A CHALLENGE?

Just as health comes with its baggage of associations, so, too, does the notion of self-care. The way I see it, self-care isn't about the list of things you are supposed to do to be healthy, or about keeping up with the new health fads or latest scientific theories. Self-care isn't about battling yourself into submission to satisfy the agendas of your inner critic.

Self-care is about a fundamental orientation toward the self that is rooted in kindness and compassion. It is about nourishing all of who you are. And at its foundation, it is about your capacity to truly love and honor yourself and your life.

As wonderful as it sounds, this is far from easy. The spiritual teacher Adyashanti often tells his students, "The person you'll have the hardest time opening to and truly loving without reserve is yourself. Once you can do that, you can love the whole universe unconditionally."[10]

So don't be surprised if self-care doesn't come naturally, or even if you have unexpected and irrational resistance to doing it. We all have baggage, wounds, traumas, and beliefs that keep us from being able to turn toward ourselves with the level of kindness, compassion, and loving care that we may easily be able to extend toward others.

Learning how to face and embrace those parts of ourselves that we have disowned, or that are weighed down in shame or self-judgment, is foundational to having an empowered relationship with our own self-care. This is something we'll be coming back to as we work our way through the Vitality Map.

Issues like shame, self-judgment, and self-sabotage are rarely talked about in conventional health circles. And yet they are critical, and we can't ignore them if we wish to discover and live in our innate vitality and thriving health. If we are unable to turn toward ourselves with loving care, how can we expect to be able to sustain life-giving habit changes?

It's also hard to follow through with something that we're not fully invested in. For example, I was recently talking with a new client who had the intention to integrate more movement into her life. She excitedly told me that she thought she had a great strategy. Since she had to be up early to take her daughter to school, she would just go straight to work and use the gym there before seeing clients. When I asked her what kinds of movement she loved to do, she listed going for long bike rides, hiking, walking with friends, and going to yoga or Pilates classes. When I pointed out that the gym wasn't on her list, she admitted that she actually hates going to the gym. We laughed about how her strategy probably wouldn't last so long! We were then able to come up with a better way to follow through on her intention for more movement by doing things she actually loves to do.

INVITING A FEMININE APPROACH

It seems to me that what has been missing in our approach to health and self-care is what many people would refer to as "the feminine." Our culture's tendency to prioritize a more masculine kind of productivity has bled into how we approach health and self-care—hence the managerial approach of getting things done, checking symptoms off the list, and making sure that we have tended to ourselves as we are supposed to. A masculine orientation prioritizes leading from the mind and relies on the use of willpower to make things happen.

This is not a negative thing in and of itself—indeed, this approach can be credited with many of the advances in modern medicine over the last few centuries, breakthroughs that have saved countless lives and improved life expectancy for all of us. But perhaps we've gone too far in that direction. It's time for a rebalancing of the masculine and feminine energies when it comes to our healthcare. This is true for both men and women. These archetypal energies are not synonymous with our physical sex or our gender. Many women, for example, still take a very masculine approach to their self-care.

Feminine energy, connected with our creativity and emergence, is more slow, fluid, intuitive, and gentle. Just as a mother holds a young child in pain, the feminine values patience, nurturing, and a loving embrace. The feminine is about receptivity and openness, and an intimate connection with one's body and emotions.

Imagine for yourself what it would be to honor and invite the feminine more fully into your self-care journey. What would that offer you? How would it change how you hold and relate to yourself? For me, it evokes questions like these throughout my days as I am faced with choices:

+ Am I being kind to myself?

+ Am I needing more self-gentleness right now?

+ What would bring me greater ease here?

+ How can I open more fully to pleasure?

By embracing the feminine in our self-care journey we can slowly, gently, playfully, and easefully learn how to honor and love ourselves into our most vibrant, alive potentials. It's an orientation of awake self-responsibility in your health journey—one that is not harsh, mean, or judgmental, but instead is rooted in love and kindness, as well as gentle, nurturing care.

CHECKING IN: *How does it feel in your body right now to imagine bringing a more feminine approach to your self-care? What does it viscerally evoke for you? What does it evoke emotionally?*

OUR MOMENT IN HISTORY

I feel for our human family at this time in history. We're in the midst of such complexity and transformation, and it can feel utterly disorienting. The impacts of the times we're living in are akin to a modern invisible plague. The realities we're navigating, individually and as a human family, are changing so rapidly. Ingenuity and creativity are soaring. Old systems are crumbling. Every day it seems we have new technologies, new demands on our time, more ways to communicate (and be inundated with messages we don't have time to return), new pressures and challenges to negotiate. We're all in it together, fumbling around as humans trying to integrate and relate to what is happening, barely getting used to one thing, when the next thing shows up.

In a very brief amount of time, we have shifted into a level of global awareness and connection that is unprecedented. It can be so hard (and perhaps impossible) to wrap our minds around the complexity of it all. Yet the psychic pressure is there in the background—the weapons of mass destruction, the loss of species, the changing face of our natural world, climate change, compromised food supplies, and so much more.

We're all taking the brunt of it, whether we realize it or not.

Even if we're not thinking about these big, global issues, even if we just focus on what is right in front of us, our daily responsibilities and realities, we can be so totally overwhelmed. There are such strong cultural priorities placed on productivity, efficiency, and keeping busy. Because we are embedded in these paradigms, and we're all navigating the rapid complexity of changes as a human species at this time in history, it feels to me like we're in an outbreak of what I've come to call the "Over-Everything Syndrome."

It shows up differently for different people, yet so many of us live with the dial turned up to high all the time. And it is almost like we have forgotten how to turn the dial down, to really let go in life, to relax and feel deeply at ease—rested, nourished, replenished. And if we do experience these precious states, it is relegated to vacation time for a couple of weeks a year. And it's not just because we don't have the opportunity. Jacqueline Olds, MD, and Richard S. Schwartz, MD, write in *The Lonely American* that "American workers gave back, or didn't take advantage of, 574 million vacation days in 2005, the equivalent of more than 20,000 lifetimes. Surveys done by Gallup and the Conference Board indicate that Americans, who already take fewer vacation days than workers in any other industrial nation in the world, are cutting back even further. About 25 percent of Americans get no paid vacation time, and another 33 percent will take only a seven-day vacation."[11]

Not surprisingly, our stress levels are off the charts. Every system in our bodies is affected. Inflammation is high. The natural feedback loops that keep us in a state of vitality and resilience exhaust themselves and no longer function properly. Our hormones, neurochemicals, and immune systems get wonky. When I look at many of the diseases that are rampant these days, it seems to me that stress is at the heart of them, or at least a strong contributor.

The American Psychological Association states that, "if untreated, consistently high stress could become a chronic condition, which can result in serious health problems including anxiety, insomnia, muscle pain, high blood pressure and a weakened immune system. Research shows that stress can even contribute to the development of major illnesses, such as heart disease, depression and obesity, or exacerbate existing illnesses."[12]

Arianna Huffington, in her book *Thrive*, shares that "according to the Centers for Disease Control and Prevention, as much as three-quarters of the country's healthcare spending goes toward treating these kinds of chronic conditions." And she cites researchers at the Benson-Henry Institute for Mind Body Medicine at Massachusetts General Hospital as estimating that between 60 and 90 percent of doctor's visits are connected to stress-related conditions.[13]

We no longer know how to turn our dials down. One of my clients, Stacy, is a physician in a three-year residency program. She commonly works seventy-plus hours per week, including alternating regularly between night and day shifts. She has reported frequently to me how hard it is for her to stop doing things even in the limited amount of time off she has, as there are always things to do—shopping, laundry, cleaning, follow-up work, studying, and residency assignments. While Stacy's schedule may be extreme, we all have our own versions of how hard it can be to let down. We no longer know how to live from a place where ease and relaxation is the foundation.

Have you ever gone on vacation or had a transitional period in your work when there was less to do and noticed how uncomfortable it can initially feel to have spaciousness and unstructured time? It can be hard to remember what to do with all of that freedom. It can even cause an increase in anxiety for many of us.

We can be so caught up in the momentum of what's happening that we lose connection with the bigger picture of our lives and what we really need to be nourishing and tending to in our own state of vitality and wellness. We are so busy being busy that we neglect ourselves in critical ways—emotionally, psychologically, spiritually, and physically.

BASIC LIFE SKILLS WE WERE NEVER TAUGHT

I see the challenges we face today in the world as a generative force, calling us all to develop the skills, capacities, and orientations we need in order to care for ourselves, each other, and the world. If this sounds like yet another task to add to your endless to-do list, don't worry. I'm not asking you to take a crash course in medicine, or to venture into the bewildering maze of online medical information. The skills I'm teaching you here are not actually "new" capacities at all—they are already in you, they may simply never have been activated. Once you start to engage with them, they will slowly but surely become natural, and the end result will be a foundation of deep ease and self-compassion that will help you get off the treadmill of modern life and find your own balance.

Many people I meet feel utterly confused about their inability to effectively care for themselves. As I shared in the previous chapter, they even feel shame and embarrassment that they ought to know better. You might wonder how you could have gotten to this point of feeling so out of touch with your ability to guide yourself toward a thriving life.

Here's where the big embrace of self-compassion begins: *It's not your fault. There is nothing wrong with you.*

You simply never learned what I consider to be basic life skills of how to intimately and confidently care for yourself. I never learned these skills either. Most people don't. I came into them through a very rocky journey of self-discovery and once I began to see them and apply them I realized how utterly ridiculous it was that I never knew how to relate to my own self-care in these ways.

I imagine you may experience this too as you engage with the 9 Keys to Deep Vitality. At times, they may seem utterly simple and obvious. And yet, the application of them is profound. These skills are what allow us to cultivate the soil of our lives and come alive to who we are here to be.

I find it to be such a relief to recognize that health is in fact about learning these basic, innate life skills we were simply never taught. Understanding this can move us out of the sense of disempowerment that so often accompanies our attempts to improve our health. Rather than seeming so mysterious and confusing, health becomes something we can consciously decide to engage with and thus we can take charge of our lives at this most fundamental level.

Investing in learning the skills and expanding your capacity to gracefully and intelligently care for yourself is like taking the time to make sure that you are building a strong, solid foundation for your house. You wouldn't want to be living in a house that had a foundation thrown together quickly and with little planning. Before long your house would be sinking and tilting sideways. You couldn't live there anymore!

Because most of us were never taught how to care for ourselves with conscious intimate awareness, knowledge, and skills related to healthy self-regulation, our health journey has lacked a foundation. We get spun around with all of the protocols, theories, and fads, trying them out with little sustained success. Without a solid foundation we're left spinning, tilting, feeling the ground beneath us to be shaky.

As you embrace and work with each of the 9 Keys to Deep Vitality, think of the process as similar to adding different layers of design and construction to your beautiful, strong, comfortable home. Your body is your home for this lifetime, housing YOU, in all of your unique, complex, subtle beauty. I like to refer to this as "body-home," a shorthand term for the particular physical, mental, emotional, spiritual dwelling that you inhabit.

The 9 Keys to Deep Vitality are vitality fundamentals that most of us were never taught. These are the skills of self-care and intimate self-knowing that can put you in direct contact with all the things that nourish your body-home into its full aliveness.

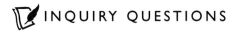 INQUIRY QUESTIONS

Before we move forward into preparing for your journey, let's take a closer look at how you're nurturing or stifling your vitality in specific areas of your life. For each of the following life aspects, please list how you are currently nourishing your vitality, as well as any specific concerns or needs for support you recognize:

+ **Mental & Emotional** (e.g., moods, perspectives, outlook, focus, motivation, presence, mental clarity, self-awareness)

+ **Physical** (e.g., energy, pain, exercise, sleep, infection, nutrition, digestion, respiration, any medical diagnoses or body systems)

+ **Personal Transformation & Development** (e.g., expanding awareness, a sense of one's own evolution and growth, curiosity, motivation)

+ **Play & Recreation** (e.g., whatever it is for you that elicits the spirit of a carefree innocent child, joy, spontaneity, FUN, relaxation)

+ **Relationships, Community, & Culture** (e.g., family, romance, friendships, sexuality, support, sense of belonging/connection, collaboration, intimacy)

+ **Spirituality & Religion** (e.g., sense of a deeper connection/greater meaning to life, soul's purpose, intuition, guiding principles/values, exploration of consciousness)

+ **Service & Work** (e.g., what you offer to the greater society, sense of fulfillment, how you generate livelihood, money/finances, security)

+ **Nature & World** (e.g., how grounded are you in nature and the other contexts of your life: environment, society, global community, politics)

CHAPTER 3

A JOURNEY INTO
DEEP HEALTH

✦

"You can trust the promise of this opening;
Unfurl yourself into the grace of beginning
That is at one with your life's desire."
—JOHN O'DONOHUE

THE PATH OF deep health is a sacred journey. "Sacred" isn't limited to religious or spiritual beliefs and practices. The word "sacred," to me, is about what connects us to the mysterious wonder in and awe of life. It is about living in a simple, direct, conscious relationship with the astonishing reality of existence. The territory through which this health journey will take you is not the outer world but your own inner landscapes. It is not a journey that can be hurried, and there are no shortcuts—it will unfold in its own time, as your inner vitality slowly matures.

Navigating the transformational terrain of health has been like a pilgrimage for me, requiring an ongoing surrender and trust in life. Although its forms vary from religion to religion, pilgrimage seems to be a recurring theme found across spiritual traditions: one goes on a long journey rooted in devotion to pay homage to a particular sacred site, or as a rite of passage, or as a quest to connect with a deeper guidance.

As author Paulo Coehlo shares in his book *The Pilgrimage*, "When you are moving toward an objective . . . it is very important to pay attention to the road. It is the road that teaches us the best way to get there, and the road enriches us as we walk its length."[14] Step by step, the walking reveals the territory. The outer world through which you travel can reflect and reveal the inner territory of your own growth and opening. Even if the journey is not what you expected at the outset, it will show you what is most essential.

Coehlo goes on to say, "When you travel, you experience, in a very practical way, the act of rebirth."[15] The journey into new territories, both inner and outer, changes you. The sacred orientation of a pilgrimage asks you to let go of who you have been and enter into a gestation of sorts. Pilgrimage, by design, opens you up in such a way that you are able to consciously embrace the gifts that transition offers. The act of walking is a metaphor for one's life, a movement of becoming, providing time to nurture a gradual emergence of a new self. Priorities and perspectives shift. Your sense of who you are and what you are capable of takes on new frames of reference outside of the cultural norms, paradigms, and assumptions you may have previously been immersed in. You may find yourself moving beyond limits that had seemed impassable before. You may feel as if you have emerged out of a small room with four walls and a low ceiling into a wide-open landscape under a vast blue sky.

The Vitality Map is your reference guide as you embark on your pilgrimage toward health. This isn't a traditional pilgrimage that is about paying homage to a sacred deity or place. It is about walking the deeper path of liberating your own well-being. In the spirit of pilgrimage, you will find that health is not an end destination—it is the journey. As you travel, you will learn to honor your own body at every step, nurturing its capacity to carry you. You will learn to be sensitive to the flow of your energy, allowing your body to rest and renew and develop the stamina and strength to continue moving forward.

The nine keys open the door to this territory, making what could be a disorienting, trying journey into one that you can gently move through. They help to reveal the new terrain, and hold you in a process and container that allows you to travel as deeply and intimately as you choose to go. They guide you into a direct, awake relationship with caring for and nourishing the most authentic, alive, vital expression of yourself. They connect you with what really matters, with the bigger picture of this life journey that you are on.

CHECKING IN: *In the spirit of pilgrimage, I ask you to stand up, set the book down, and walk around for a minute as you allow the ideas in this chapter to give rise to physical sensations, thoughts, and feelings that naturally want to emerge.*

As you move through this book and apply the keys in your own life, you will begin to consciously author a new health story. At times I imagine you may find yourself resting with a level of ease and vital life-energy that you have never known before, empowered in your capacity to guide yourself with conscious care and radical self-knowing. At other times, however, it may feel uncomfortable, like you were a pilgrim caught out in the cold rain with many miles still to travel that day. At moments like this, I hope you will remember to honor the fact that you are in transition. Something beautiful is readying itself to be born.

As Stephen Pressfield eloquently writes in *The War of Art,* "When we conceive of an enterprise and commit to it in the face of our fears, something wonderful happens. A crack appears in the membrane. Like the first craze when a chick pecks at the inside of its shell. Angel midwives congregate around us; they assist as we give birth to ourselves, to that person we were born to be, to the one whose destiny was encoded in our soul."[16]

Through all of the ups and downs, I'll be here as intimately, and with as much presence, as I can be through the words on these pages, holding you on your path. I'll be offering you a map of the territory for this sacred pilgrimage of health, opening up the space for you to stay in your life-giving movement. And I'll be here encouraging you to continue to come back to a self-loving embrace, to trust in the process, and to commit deeply to steering yourself toward your own thriving.

Before we begin, let's survey the territory.

THE 9 KEYS TO DEEP VITALITY: AN OVERVIEW

I find it a reassuring and grounding experience to take in the broad overview of the territory that I am about to explore, even if I can't predict what will emerge during the journey itself. The Vitality Map is the big-picture perspective on the landscape of health you are about to venture into.

Within each of the 9 Keys to Deep Vitality you'll find various dynamic practices offered to support you in shifting out of an intellectual engagement and into a felt experience and integration into your daily life. This framework, each key building on the next, will allow you to engage closely with the material to make it intimately relevant to who you uniquely are and to the realities of your daily life.

KEY #1: HONORING YOUR UNIQUE LIFE

You are the only one who can transform your health and find a path that will sustain you in the long run. Doctors can help. Friends can help. Family can help. But only you hold the keys to make your life blossom, flourish, and thrive.

KEY #2: FACING AND EMBRACING YOUR SHADOWS

The main obstacles to deep health and vitality are the unconscious thought patterns, assumptions, and other shadow aspects that sabotage even your best intentions to change. When you illuminate and embrace these shadows, you free your capacity to sustain the transformation you seek.

KEY #3: STRENGTHENING YOUR SELF-AWARENESS MUSCLES

In order to become a conscious steward of your own vitality, you need to learn the art of receiving feedback from your body. Your body will tell you what it needs, and as you learn to heed its messages, you become your own best health guide.

KEY #4: CULTIVATING RESILIENCE

Most of us were never taught how to guide ourselves toward actions, attitudes, and practices that support rather than hinder our own vitality. Learn to cultivate your capacity to direct yourself in more nourishing directions with discernment, skillfulness, and confidence.

KEY #5: ALIGNING WITH YOUR "YES!"

Discover how to consciously invest your life-energy where you get the best returns, letting go of those things that inhibit your natural and organic blossoming.

KEY #6: EXPERIMENTING WITH PLAYFUL CURIOSITY

Free yourself from the trap of being too serious about health and self-care—all of the rights and wrongs, the shoulds and shouldn'ts. Learn to be flexible, curious, and playful on your health journey so that you can sustain it in the long run.

KEY #7: DISCOVERING EASEFUL DISCIPLINE

In order to sustain the changes you seek, you sometimes need clear commitments, intelligent strategies, and structures of support. This kind of discipline springs from a dedication to honoring your unique life—fierce, yet full of compassion.

KEY #8: INVITING SUPPORT AND CONNECTION

No ingredient is more powerful and essential than developing relationships that will support you in your health journey. You can't do it alone. We all need each other.

KEY #9: LIVING LIKE YOU MATTER

Your health isn't just about you. It is the foundation that you need to serve the world. You are a vital member of life. Our world needs you! You need you. You matter.

PREPARING FOR THE JOURNEY

In the ritualistic work that I've done, leading mini vision-quest wilderness journeys as well as working with my clients and groups in other programs, I have come to be a huge proponent of the power of clarifying and naming our intentions and commitments at the beginning of the journey.

I have seen time and again that taking the time to engage in a conscious process of commitment serves to root you on your authentic path. It brings a potency of engagement that anchors you in the larger picture of your life, of what really matters, of what this journey is really about for you.

While the journey will continue to deepen and clarify what you only have a mere glimpse of now, finding the courage to step in with your whole being and align with your intentions and commitments will carry you forward.

The territory revealed in the Vitality Map is one that you can deepen into for the rest of your life. Even if you skate through the map quickly, you will find tips and techniques to take with you as you move forward in your life. My hope is that you will choose to dive deep. It is what is down beneath the surface that will result in the lifelong transformation and healing. That's the terrain that I find the most rewards in, the most transformative energies, and it is my dearest wish that you will feel held and guided there in the pages that follow.

In the first two chapters, I offered journaling exercises designed to help you see with clear eyes your current landscape of health and your relationship with your self-care. Now that you have begun to get a bit of a taste of the terrain ahead, I offer the following questions to help guide you in clarifying your intentions and commitments.

Before you open your journal to write, I'd like to invite you to pause, close your eyes, and connect with the felt sensations of your body. As you feel yourself becoming more present to the moment and to your feelings, see if you can drop down and listen for that inner guidance and life wisdom, that voice or sense within that alerts you to what is in alignment with your own thriving and what is not.

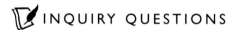

INQUIRY QUESTIONS

Give yourself some time to journal using the following questions as inspiration:

- ✦ What intentions do I have for embarking on this journey, guided by the Vitality Map?

- ✦ What am I yearning to receive and learn?

- ✦ What am I willing to give to this experience?

- ✦ What are my life priorities? What am I committed to now, above all else?

Once you have finished writing your answers, I would strongly encourage you to share them with someone you trust, someone who can hold the sacredness and vulnerability of this journey with you. By having someone trustworthy and loving listen to your intentions and commitments, you may find it easier to embody those intentions and commitments, to connect and stay true to them. They will become real. Perhaps you might even invite a friend or loved one along with you on this journey—someone who you know is ripe to dive deep in the same ways that you are. Together you can create an ongoing path of mutual sharing, learning, growing, and healing.

9 KEYS TO
DEEP VITALITY

KEY #1: HONORING YOUR UNIQUE LIFE

KEY #2: FACING AND EMBRACING YOUR SHADOWS

KEY #3: STRENGTHENING YOUR SELF-AWARENESS MUSCLES

KEY #4: CULTIVATING RESILIENCE

KEY #5: ALIGNING WITH YOUR YES!

KEY #6: EXPERIMENTING WITH PLAYFUL CURIOSITY

KEY #7: DISCOVERING EASEFUL DISCIPLINE

KEY #8: INVITING SUPPORT AND CONNECTION

KEY #9: LIVING LIKE YOU MATTER

HONORING YOUR UNIQUE LIFE

"The privilege of a lifetime is being who you are."
—JOSEPH CAMPBELL

HAVE YOU EVER come close to death? Have you ever seen a baby being born? Have you lost a loved one unexpectedly? Have you stood looking at a glorious sunset, a mountain vista, or a starry sky and felt overcome by awe and gratitude? All of these experiences, whether joyful or painful, have one thing in common: they bring us in touch with the beauty and preciousness of life. For a moment, often a fleeting one, we become conscious of the gift of being here, in our bodies, on this rich and life-sustaining planet, surrounded by people we love.

What also often happens in such moments is that we realize how we have been living unconsciously—sleepwalking through our days, unaware of the fragility and significance of our human incarnation. We "wake up" to the wonder of it all and swear to ourselves that we will never again allow ourselves to forget or take for granted this extraordinary life.

But we do. When the heightened intensity of joy, or grief, or wonder fades, most of us go back to being out of touch with that sense of gratitude, value, and sacredness of our lives. And particularly when it comes to caring for our fragile human bodies, we rarely remember to treat them with the respect and honor that they deserve.

The first of the nine keys, Honoring Your Unique Life, is about connecting to a sense of reverence and responsibility for your own body, your own soul, and your own unique spark of the miracle of life. I don't want you to have to wait until some unexpected tragedy or moment of inspiration puts you in touch with that feeling. You can access it right now, if you simply contemplate what it means to be you, to be here, to be alive.

🎧 **GUIDED MEDITATION**: *Let's pause for a moment and allow this recognition of the incredible gift of your life to emerge. You may want to close your eyes and imagine that you are becoming conscious of your body for the very first time. With the curiosity and wonder of a young child let your awareness notice all the subtle sensations that are indicating that you are alive right now. Feel the vital life-energy coursing through you, breathing you, pumping your blood through your veins. Check in with each of your senses—what are you smelling, hearing, tasting, feeling, and seeing right now? Acknowledge how amazing it is to be able to hear the birds singing outside, to taste the sweetness of your favorite tea, to see the blue of the sky, to smell the scent of fresh-cut grass. Notice the thoughts and feelings moving through your consciousness and recognize the astonishing capacity of your mental and emotional intelligence. Allow yourself to sink even deeper and connect with the silent stillness that lies beneath all the layers of who you are. And then take a moment to appreciate the miraculous fact that you are able to be consciously aware of all of this.*

As environmental activist and ecologist Joanna Macy so eloquently says, "To be alive in this beautiful, self-organizing universe—to participate in the dance of life with senses to perceive it, lungs that breathe it, organs that draw nourishment from it—is a wonder beyond words."[17]

I know it can be incredibly easy to take being alive for granted. And yet when I stop and consciously guide myself into a heightened awareness of my life, I am often dumbstruck by how utterly, incomprehensibly extraordinary it all is. No matter what your religious, spiritual, or scientific leanings may be, I wonder if you feel it, too—the incredible miracle of being alive, the awe-inspiring fact that you are utterly unique? You are the only you there is and will ever be!

If the awareness of your unique and precious life is hard to access, or if it is not a feeling that is familiar to you, this may be a moment to stop and reflect on how you are moving through your days.

One of my clients, Andrea, described to me how she reached a point where she was "just living on autopilot." Approaching fifty, divorced, overweight, and with the prospect of an empty nest looming as her youngest prepared to go to college, she said, "I guess the best way I can describe it is that my life is just happening to me. I don't change anything in my days. I get up because I have to be somewhere or I have to do something. I go to my job and just work through my to-do list. And then I go home. I'm not present, and nothing brings me joy. I sometimes think that if I were to die tomorrow that would be totally fine with me because I've had a decent life and I guess this is all there is."

I told Andrea how much I appreciated her honesty and vulnerability in sharing this, and assured her she was not at all alone in feeling that way. "I also know that you wouldn't be here if there weren't part of you that wanted to feel alive and awake to your life again," I told her. As I said those words Andrea nodded and began to gently cry. I continued, "You've made a really powerful choice to step into a new level of self-responsibility for nourishing yourself."

As soon as I said the word—"responsibility"—I saw her face shut down. For a moment I wished I'd chosen a different word, to spare her all the reactions and associations she clearly had, but then I thought again. After all, it was the right word. And if Andrea was going to turn her life around, it was going to be essential for her to find a new way of relating to the word "responsibility."

If you, too, had a reaction to that word, that's great. I find that facing things directly can lead us to a deeper truth much more quickly. I like to help reveal what's really going on, and our instinctive reactions are sometimes the very signposts that can lead us to the truth. While it is uncomfortable (sometimes profoundly so!), I find it empowering to look at things as they are, and not sugarcoat them. In my experience, this is the pathway to freedom, the freedom we need to create something different for ourselves. So let's look at what the word "responsibility" triggers in relation to your own self-care.

📝 INQUIRY QUESTIONS

Write down the word "responsibility" in your journal, or say it out loud to yourself, and then ask:

✦ What associations do I have with responsibility?

✦ What visceral reactions arise in my body?

✦ What does it feel like emotionally for me?

For Andrea, it brought up the voice of her inner critic. "When you say 'responsibility,'" she admitted, "I just feel the part of me that is already constantly berating myself for not being good enough. I feel my whole body tensing up and my emotions shutting down. I've done that for years—striving to never make a mistake, to look perfect, to eat healthy, to work the hardest, to be the best. That's how I made myself crazy."

As we continued to explore her experience, Andrea admitted that there was another side to her relationship to responsibility. "I also have a rebellious part of me—it almost feels like a rebellion against my own body. I'll defy all the rules and regulations that my mind is constantly imposing on me, and instead I'll eat and drink to excess and not exercise. I don't let anyone see this—on the outside there is control, but on the inside there is rebellion."

THE REBELLIOUS TEENAGER
AND THE STRICT ADULT

These two responses that Andrea described reflect patterns I've observed time and time again in myself and my adult clients when it comes to taking responsibility in relationship to our own health journey. I've summarized them as two "characters"—the Rebellious Teenager and the Strict Adult.

THE REBELLIOUS TEENAGER: Some of us get triggered into feeling like a thirteen-year-old rebel when it comes to responsibility for our own self-care. We tune out. We look away. We stop reading. We don't even want to hear the word "responsibility," because it's no fun, and we just associate it with this whole external list of things that we *should* be doing. All of those "rights" and "wrongs." It feels like a burden and it's what we hate about being adults. We tend toward avoidance, as well as self-sabotage, in response to the way we know deep down we ought to be attending to ourselves.

THE STRICT ADULT: Others of us identify a great deal with *being responsible*. We've created our sense of self, the structures of who we are and how we show up in the world, around being a responsible person. We bolster ourselves up for being accountable and getting things done or make ourselves feel bad if we don't live up to our ideals and rules. Our identity and sense of self-worth is wrapped up in being responsible. We've adopted an orientation of "managing" ourselves in all the ways we are "supposed to," in order to be healthy. Yet we may be aware that we easily become tightly strung as a result. Or we feel stressed out all the time. Or we don't seem able to play and let loose like we yearn to, or we may even feel like we've forgotten how to live that way. While we might be doing what we "should" be doing, thriving health and vitality still seem to elude us.

In my experience, most of us find ourselves swinging back and forth across this spectrum. We rebel against ourselves after being very diligent and strict for a certain period. We are unable to find a sense of ease regardless of which side of the conundrum we fall. This is a classic "boom and bust" cycle in relationship to self-care.

In the course of my own health journey, I have seen myself all over that spectrum. For years I bounced back and forth between rigid self-management and rebellious self-neglect, until eventually I found my way to an entirely new orientation to responsibility for my own self-care.

Looking back on that time now, I have so much compassion for my younger self. I'm grateful to have experienced how fully life brought me to my knees, and to have been able to live through the spectrum of human responses to my own health crisis. While I would not wish unnecessary suffering on myself or on anyone, I doubt that I could have come to the new understandings that created the approach I share with my clients and in the pages of this book without having lived through what I have.

YOUR SECRET SUPERPOWER

Here's what I've come to know: We're not all doomed to forever play out the strict/rebellious—or boom-and-bust—cycles in relationship to our own self-care. There is another way of embracing responsibility that is outside of that paradigm.

As I shared with Andrea, this key to vitality, Honoring Your Unique Life, starts with recognizing these habitual inner patterns in ourselves. For her, it was a revelation. She later told me, "When you introduced the two person-alities—the Strict Adult and the Rebellious Teenager—in such a way that I could name them, that was a really big shift for me. When I was falling into one or the other, I could feel it and know what I was going through, instead of just being in this whirlwind of patterns I didn't understand."

She also acknowledged the importance of starting to listen to a new and different part of herself and with the help of that new part, find her own way. "I remember, at the beginning, that I kept trying to get you to give me rules and regulations!" she recalled, laughing. "You didn't tell me how I needed to change or all of the steps to take. Instead you would help me to really feel what was going on and to face and get underneath the self-talk. You would gently, gently guide me and I would just keep talking, and it was almost like you were letting me come up with the things that made sense for me instead of trying to change me. If I had been working with another practitioner, with someone who gave me rules and boundaries and guide-lines, I'm sure my inner Strict Adult would have taken those and tried to be the best patient they ever had. And it would have turned it into more of my disease, instead of helping me heal."

What Andrea learned was to access a deeper source of inner guidance and wisdom that was rooted in consciously acknowledging the gift of her life. Her orientation to her own self-care radically shifted. Her new sense of responsibility was born not from guilt, shame, or what she thought she was supposed to do, but from honor, respect, and gratitude. In other words, she came to experience a sense of reverence for her own life. And please let me assure you that there is nothing narcissistic or overtly religious about this. This is about recognizing that you have received the incredible gift and blessing of being alive—whether you believe it comes from God or from evolution or even just from random chance.

These words, from physician and clinical professor Rachel Naomi Re-men, resonate deeply for me, as they capture what this first key, Honoring Your Unique Life, is all about:

The real truth is that Self-Care is a practice that can draw us closer to the sanctity of life. If we do not recognize and value the life in our own selves, how can we learn to value the life in others? Integrity, in its sim-plest yet most profound form, requires that our intention toward life be coherent and whole and that we each practice being harmless and compassionate—not only toward the life in others but also toward the life that is uniquely our own.[18]

That leads us to the heart of it all: the natural, humbling acknowledgment that caring for ourselves is at the very foundation of our service to life. We each are here to support and encourage the fullness of our own exquisitely unique, vital life expression. Why? Because no one else is here to do that. We are each born into that job, that innate responsibility. And it is only when we disconnect from the gratitude and reverence for, as the poet Mary Oliver puts it, our "one wild and precious life"[19] that this feels like a burden.

I love the way the great dancer Martha Graham famously described that unique, vital life expression, in a letter to her longtime friend and confidante Cecil B. DeMille:

There is a vitality, a life force, an energy, a quickening, that is translated through you into action, and because there is only one of you in all time, this expression is unique. And if you block it, it will never exist through any other medium and will be lost. The world will not have it. It is not your business to determine how good it is nor how valuable nor how it compares with other expressions. It is your business to keep it yours clearly and directly, to keep the channel open.[20]

This recognition, for me, was a turning point in my own healing journey. When I began rooting my relationship with self-care in the awe and deep gratitude for the miraculous gift of being alive, and feeling responsible for that, everything shifted. I was no longer caught up in unhealthy patterns around self-responsibility. Instead, in cultivating this awareness, this re-membrance, I became softer with myself. Gentler. More patient. It felt like I truly was able to love myself, unconditionally, for the first time.

Now, that doesn't mean that the self-judgments, shame, or demanding and critical voices just went away. They didn't. But what did happen was that other voices gained strength and volume inside, and with practice I was able to consciously choose to listen to their guidance instead.

Archetypally, it felt like I was learning to mother myself—to nurture, respect, love, and support myself in becoming who I am here to be. In other words, I came to know what it felt like to truly "have my own back." When

I feel this quality in myself, I think of it as my inner Mama Bear. She's like a secret super power! Nothing's going to get between her and her cubs, just like nothing's going to get in the way of me honoring my unique life. The fierce commitment and gentle embrace of the Mama Bear is grounded in unconditional, loving, compassionate, and nurturing care. This is an absolutely essential element of your journey to health.

Can you feel the difference between the kind of responsibility for and stewardship of yourself that comes from your inner Mama Bear versus the inner Strict Adult or Rebellious Teenager? The Mama Bear doesn't berate you with all of the rights, wrongs, and shoulds that "trying to be healthy" has become for so many of us. But neither does she rebel and neglect your health. She bypasses that whole cycle and always stands *with* you, fiercely, loyally, and lovingly, reminding you, in no uncertain terms, that your thriving matters.

INQUIRY QUESTIONS

Here's another inquiry process to help you visualize and get in touch with your inner Mama Bear. In your journal, or just in quiet contemplation, think about these questions:

+ How does a Mama Bear care for her cubs? What does she do when someone comes near her cubs? What does she do when she feels safe and like there is no threat? How does she respond when her cubs are doing something that might hurt them?

+ Imagine you have an inner Mama Bear. What are her superpowers? If you imagine that she is caring for you, as she would her cubs, what would that look like? How might she care for you in ways that you haven't been able to care for yourself?

+ How can you embrace this Mama Bear energy in how you relate to your own self-care, so that she becomes part of you? How might this help you to step out of the dance between an inner Strict Adult and a Rebellious Teenager?

For Andrea, discovering her inner Mama Bear was an important step, because she recognized that although she was a loving and nurturing parent to her kids, she'd never experienced being nurtured herself. "Treating myself as I would want my children to be treated was a huge shift," she says. "I would never be harsh or mean to my children if they were trying something new, yet I talked to myself that harshly every minute of every day. I knew they deserved unconditional love and support, but I never even considered that I did." Andrea began to have conversations with her Mama Bear in her head, and that gentle, compassionate voice became stronger than the other voices that had driven her crazy for so long.

This transformation calls to mind the words of the feminist author and social activist bell hooks:

In an ideal world we would all learn in childhood to love ourselves. We would grow, being secure in our worth and value, spreading love wherever we went, letting our light shine. If we did not learn self-love in our youth, there is still hope. The light of love is always in us, no matter how cold the flame. It is always present, waiting for the spark to ignite, waiting for the heart to awaken and call us back to the first memory of being the life force inside a dark place waiting to be born—waiting to see the light.[21]

With that "light of love" now lit within her, and fueled by her newfound commitment and self-respect, Andrea no longer feels like she's living on autopilot. She's living consciously, creatively, and with increasing joy. In fact, she surprises even herself with the unexpected choices she's making, like taking a recent trip to Hawaii with a group of friends and being the one who initiated a zip-line adventure!

CHECKING IN: *Pause now and invite your awareness into your body. What are these stories and perspectives evoking in you? How does it feel to embrace the knowledge that you alone are responsible for your unique and precious life? What does it mean to you to honor your unique life?*

YOU ARE MORTAL

Honoring your unique life necessitates confronting your mortality, being in direct relationship with how fleeting your life really is. As Bernie Siegel, MD, puts it, "An awareness of one's mortality can lead you to wake up and live an authentic, meaningful life."[22]

Research shows that people who have had near-death experiences tend to report "greater appreciation for life, a renewed sense of purpose, greater confidence and flexibility in coping with life's vicissitudes, increased value of love and service and decreased concern with personal status and material possessions, greater compassion for others, a heightened sense of spiritual purpose, and a greatly reduced fear of death."[23] And yet despite hearing stories like these, most of us spend lifetimes denying the truth of our mortality, until we reach a point where it is forced upon us.

One afternoon at school during my naturopathic medical training, rumors were spreading through the halls: one of our own, a twenty-five-year-old student in her second year, had been hit by a truck while she was biking home, and was killed instantly. I still feel a chill move through my body when I think of it. I didn't know her personally, yet I felt the impact deeply. I biked back and forth to school every day. It could easily have been me and not her. I went home that night and wrote heartfelt notes to friends and family. I cried with friends. I told everyone I loved them and shared things that I had been meaning to share. I felt the loss and fear poignantly in me every time I rode my bicycle for about a month. My daily life took on greater meaning and intensity.

This wasn't the first time I had experienced this, nor the last. Sometimes a confrontation with mortality can be brought on by a grave diagnosis, or by a near-miss, or even by a moment of heightened risk. I had another similar experience when hiking in the mountains on a trail with a steep drop-off where I knew that if I lost my balance, it would likely be the end for me.

Regardless of what brings it on, confronting our mortality gives us, for a brief time, a sense of a potent connection with how fleeting and unpredictable life really is. And with that recognition there often comes a willingness to prioritize what really matters, to be present to the precious miracle of being alive in a physical body.

Think about this for yourself. Have you ever had an experience in which you almost died and afterward viewed your life differently? Or perhaps navigating the death of a loved one, or knowing someone who died unexpectedly, brought up an awareness of your own fragility that felt especially potent?

INQUIRY QUESTIONS

Choose one of these experiences, or an experience, however small, that it conjures up from your past, and then take some time to answer the following questions in your journal:

+ What happened for you? Describe in detail what it felt like physically in your body, and emotionally. What did you do right afterward and how were you feeling? Did it affect how you related to others?

+ What awoke in you? What intentions, focus, or clarity emerged?

+ What realizations did you have about your life and what really matters to you?

GARDENING YOURSELF

The late Gabrielle Roth, author, dancer, and music/theater director, writes, "Each soul is unique, and we are called upon to break out of the minimum security prison of conformity and mediocrity to experience our soul's true magic and power. Like a plant, it needs to be nurtured to grow and blossom, and to be freed from the entangling, obscuring weeds that tend to take over."[24] In the spirit of this quotation, I will leave you with one final analogy—one that you might find particularly resonant if you're someone who loves to tend your garden and watch things grow. But whether or not you have ever gardened (or even like gardening!), I invite you to play along with me here as I take you on a guided visualization journey. You may want to also use your journal to engage with some of the questions I'll be asking.

I'd like you to imagine that you are a gardener in the spring. You have a plot of land that is yours to tend. You head outside to assess what you need to do to prepare your beds for planting this year. You remove mulch, weed, loosen up the soil, and add compost and other amendments. When you plant your seeds, you water them each day, watching carefully for that magical emergence as they sprout and push their way through the soil. You tend to those small plants, supporting them in their growth through weeding and adding the compost and nutrients they need in their growth cycle. And if they start to wither, turn color, or show signs of disease, you investigate, offer the missing ingredients, or remove what was harmful.

You show up without judgment, in service, doing what is necessary to support the natural life expression of each of the plants. They each grow and evolve in their own way, and all you are doing is providing them with what they need to thrive. That essential life-energy that causes the seed to sprout and push through the soil is an intrinsic intelligence that is expressed uniquely in each plant, creature, and being. And that same innate vitality and life-force is in you. In a sense, the archetype of the gardener embodies the ideal of serving life itself, supporting the life-energy so that it can flourish in all its various unique forms.

What if you became a gardener of yourself? What if embracing responsibility for your health meant recognizing that your role is to tend to, nourish, and love yourself into the vital life expression that *you* are here to be?

You plant yourself in contexts in which you will thrive. You take into your body a blend of nourishment that you mix up especially for yourself. You remove things that are harmful or suppressing your growth. You rejoice in caring for yourself, in witnessing your natural growth and evolution, the vibrant unique life expression that you are here to be. As a gardener of yourself, you feel the privilege that it is to nurture yourself so that you blossom, bloom, and shine out in the world as fully as possible. You are adding your beauty, your brilliance, your unique gifts and expression out into the larger garden of life.

And the "crop" you are tending, your own life, is the most precious thing there is. If you can imagine how a conscious farmer will do whatever it takes to support their crops in flourishing because their food source and livelihood depend on the health of those plants, it can help to put into perspective how the same is true for your own life. Nothing is more foundational than this.

INQUIRY QUESTIONS

✦ Can you feel the potential here to relax with ease into your innate responsibility, where you are nourishing and *allowing* your natural flourishing to happen?

✦ How would this shift the source of your life priorities?

✦ What would it mean to live in the recognition that you are the gardener of yourself, here to help your unique expression of life to blossom, flourish, and thrive?

KEY #2

FACING AND EMBRACING
YOUR SHADOWS

"It's hard to fight an enemy who has outposts in your head."
—SALLY KEMPTON

HAVE YOU EVER been confused about why you continue to repeat a be-havior that you know isn't serving you, that perhaps is even doing outright harm? Have you ever wondered why you may avoid doing the very things that you know make you feel healthy and alive? Are you tired of the boom-and-bust cycle in your self-care journey and confused about why you can't sustain the changes you seek?

I have seen it in myself, and I have certainly seen it in my clients and loved ones. Most of us are riddled with confusion, shame, and self-judgments in relation to our health journey. From what I've seen it doesn't matter how smart you are, how spiritually enlightened, how motivated and effective you can be in other parts of your life, or what image you present to the world. Inside, the voices are incessant. Whether it is the fat on your thighs, the coffee that hides your exhaustion, your secret addiction to ice cream, the insomnia that plagues you at night, or your avoidance of exercise, the voices inside will always tell you that you ought to know better and do better.

In Key #1 we came to see the connection between honoring your unique life and a self-responsibility that is rooted in a feeling much like a mother's love. Yet it is one thing to recognize that, and it is another thing to actually live it, day to day.

The reasons for your perceived failings may not be what you think. People come to me all the time with self-judgmental conclusions about why they are failing to stick to the diets, exercise regimes, and other behaviors that they know can be life-giving for them. Some of the most common ones I hear are:

"I'm lazy."

"I'm just not disciplined enough."

"I don't have what it takes."

"It doesn't seem to matter what I do, nothing changes."

"I can never seem to find the time."

However, what I've found is that these are rarely the real reasons. Unconscious parts of ourselves are operating all the time that are feeding our resistance and avoidance, encouraging self-sabotage, and creating competing commitments that we're totally unconscious of.

This key, Facing and Embracing Your Shadows, is what clears the ground for the rest of the keys to really take root in you. Why? Because our patterns of avoidance and self-sabotage have their roots in our shadows.

GETTING TO KNOW YOUR SHADOW

What I mean by shadows are those aspects of ourselves that are not in our conscious awareness. Essentially, they are the parts of ourselves that we have unconsciously disowned, repressed, or rejected.

The term "shadow," in the way I'm using it, comes from Jungian psychology. C. G. Jung, a Swiss psychiatrist and psychotherapist who founded analytical psychology, saw the psyche as containing several personified elements that interact with one another. He defined the shadow as "that hidden, repressed, for the most part inferior and guilt-laden personality whose ultimate ramifications reach back into the realm of our animal ancestors."[25] In other words, the shadow is the material that has been repressed from consciousness—such as desires, impulses, tendencies, memories, and experiences that we feel are incompatible with the persona we want to project in the world or is unacceptable to society or others.

Take my client Evelyn, for example. She grew up in a household where anger was never allowed to be expressed. She was always the smiley, content "good girl." It wasn't until she began working with me in her mid-thirties that she was able to recognize, feel, and embrace anger for herself and to see clearly how she had been repressing it all of these years.

My client Steven was sexually abused as a child. It is only now, at age sixty-two, that he is beginning to see how, because he repressed his own sexual feelings as a result of those traumatic experiences, he has never been able to truly open himself intimately with women, despite having been married twice.

Our shadows, by their nature, are things that we can't see clearly in ourselves, yet they often leave us clues to their presence. If you are wondering what some of your own shadows may be, here are some signs that might point the way to help you further uncover what is going on in "the shadows" for you:

REACTIONS TO OTHER PEOPLE: It can be so much easier to see things in other people than in ourselves. Our reactions are a great entry point to begin to reveal the shadows within. If there are things that you dislike a lot in another person, perhaps even feel repulsed by, there is likely a reflection of a part of yourself that you may not have owned and integrated. If you get into an argument with someone and are sure that you are "right," there may be an aspect of what the other person is standing for that you have rejected in yourself. Likewise, if you find yourself jealous of an attribute that someone else has, or are putting someone else on a pedestal for being extremely gifted in a particular way, you may not be seeing how you, too, have those beautiful qualities.

SELF-SABOTAGING AND AVOIDANCE BEHAVIORS: The ways in which we may be subtly (or not so subtly) numbing or causing harm to ourselves is ripe territory to explore as an entry point to the shadows. I often ask my clients who describe patterns of overeating, drinking to excess, or other addictive tendencies, "What are you really hungry for?" Through patterns like these, we can be unconsciously trying to meet real needs we have but are not in touch with (hint: oftentimes we are really hungry for connection, love, and a sense of belonging in our lives). Oftentimes there are feelings that are wanting to be acknowledged and felt and we don't know how. Evelyn, for example, was really angry, yet anger was something that "wasn't allowed," so she stuffed it down and channeled that energy into working long hours. She climbed high up the professional ladder, and yet became completely exhausted; it wasn't until she began to release and express the anger that had become a shadow that her energy began to return. The behaviors can be a clue and doorway into knowing that you are ripe for a shadow exploration.

FOLLOW THE RESISTANCE!

This is incredibly vulnerable, tender, and scary territory, and it feels important, before we go further into the chapter, to explicitly name and bring attention to the resistance that is right there at the heart of shadow work. I know there may be some of you reading who may already be tempted to skip ahead. You may feel the resistance rising up inside of you, offering you all sorts of clever reasons why this doesn't apply to you, or why you need to put the book down now and do something else. Resistance is an intimate friend to our shadows. It is almost as if it is resistance's job to try to get us to not face and embrace our shadows, to turn away from the vulnerability and keep the unconscious in our unconscious. So in a strange, paradoxical way, our resistance can actually guide us toward the shadow territory we most need to address to free ourselves.

I love how Steven Pressfield describes this in his book *The War of Art*: "Most of us have two lives. The life we live, and the unlived life within us. Between the two stands Resistance. . . . We can navigate by Resistance, letting it guide us to that calling or action that we must follow before all others. Rule of thumb: The more important a call or action is to our soul's evolution, the more Resistance we will feel toward pursuing it."[26] I'd like to urge you, no matter how daunting or uncomfortable this topic may feel, to stay with me here. This is truly your pathway to freedom and wholeness.

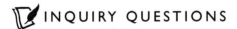 INQUIRY QUESTIONS

Here are some questions you could explore in your journal to begin uncovering places where your shadow might be hiding:

+ In what aspects of your self-care do you experience the most avoidance, resistance, or self-sabotaging patterns? How do you block your own thriving?

+ When do these patterns flare up for you? Are you able to see any correlations with other things going on in your life? In your work, in your home life, when you are feeling particular emotions?

✦ If you take a moment and open yourself to that deep place of self-knowing and really listen, what does that knowing place tell you? What is
really going on underneath your patterns?

Because we tend to reject or repress the least desirable aspects of our personalities, the shadow is largely negative. Some people see it as wholly negative, and even equate it with evil. However, Jung acknowledged that there
can also be positive aspects that remain hidden in one's shadow. For example, people with low self-esteem may repress or deny their own strengths.
"If it has been believed hitherto that the human shadow was the source of
evil, it can now be ascertained on closer investigation that the unconscious
man . . . does not consist only of morally reprehensible tendencies, but also
displays a number of good qualities, such as normal instincts, appropriate
reactions, realistic insights, creative impulses etc."[27]

The shadow is most problematic when it is unrecognized. As Jungian
analyst Christopher Perry writes, "[Jung] saw quite clearly that failure to
recognise, acknowledge and deal with shadow elements is often the root of
problems between individuals and within groups and organisations." The
reason for this is that as humans, we have a tendency to project our unwant-
ed qualities onto others or to become dominated by the shadow without
realizing it.

As Marianne Williamson writes, "Until we have met the monsters in
ourselves, we keep trying to slay them in the outer world. And we find
that we cannot. For all darkness in the world stems from darkness in the
heart. And it is there that we must do our work."[28] The shadow can cause
trouble not just in our relationships with others, but in our relationship
with ourselves. As this key will make clear, shadow issues are often at the
root of our self-sabotaging patterns and unhealthy habits. In his book *The
Divided Mind,* mind-body medicine pioneer Dr. John E. Sarno, a professor
at New York University School of Medicine, writes about how repressed or
unconscious emotions can give rise to physical symptoms (known as psy-
chosomatic disorders), and argues that the purpose of such symptoms is "to
deliberately distract the conscious mind . . . diverting attention from what is
transpiring in the unconscious."[29] Or, as the writer Anaïs Nin put it, "When
one is pretending, the entire body revolts."[30]

The more we can make conscious our shadow, the less it can dominate
us and trip us up. But remember, the shadow is an integral part of human

nature, and the idea that it can ever be eliminated only reinforces its tendency to stay hidden.

You may be completely new to the idea of shadow work, or you may have
already done a great deal with a therapist or a spiritual teacher. If you have
explored this before, you know the kind of courage and dedication it takes
to reveal aspects of yourself that have not been in your conscious awareness.
It can be incredibly humbling, surprising, and disorienting.

If you have done shadow work before, I can imagine you have felt some
benefits in your life of feeling more whole, more at home with the complexity of all of who you are. And yet you may still see yourself playing out the
kinds of self-sabotaging patterns in relation to your health that I outlined
above.

Here's what I've noticed in many people I've worked with: the shadow
work they have done has not been linked consciously with their relationship
with self-care. Beautiful healing may have been happening on one level of
themselves, but without the full integration. For instance, you may have a
wonderful revealing session with your therapist and then spend the next
two weeks binging on foods that make you feel bad. When we weave our
exploration of shadows into the very foundation of how we relate with and
care for ourselves in our daily lives, an opportunity arises for greater integration and wholeness for all of us.

IT *IS* A BIG DEAL

Lisa, a forty-nine-year-old business manager with two grown children, had
struggled with her weight all of her adult life. "I spent huge amounts of
time on weight issues—thinking about how much should I eat, how much
shouldn't I eat, 'oh I ate that, I shouldn't have,' 'I should starve myself.'
Changing diets every single day in my head, sometimes even hourly. Just
constant talk about what I'm not doing, what I should be doing. It never,
ever stopped. And I could never stick to anything. Now, I just come home,
drink, and fall into bed and get up and do the same thing over and over
and over."

As Lisa described her patterns, I felt certain the shadow was at play. She
was clearly miserable, and she'd tried everything, but she kept sabotaging
her own progress, and then using food and alcohol to numb out the emo-

tional pain. She isolated herself and pushed others away.

I asked her to tell me about her childhood. As she spoke, the pieces started to fall into place. Her mother had been sick and never fully available for her when she was young. Her father was harsh, militant, and an alcoholic. Lisa downplayed the pain of these early years, but I could hear it beneath the words as she said, "I learned my lessons my dad's way, harshly." She developed survival strategies, and one of those was to hide all signs of weakness. Other people were not to be trusted, she learned. Her shadow contained all the things she perceived as negative—vulnerability, openness, trust, connection.

She was clearly uncomfortable even talking to me about it. "Look, it's no big deal," she insisted, wanting to move on. But I knew that because this was the area in which she felt most uncomfortable it was the very place she needed to go if she were to break out of the unhealthy cycles that were stealing her happiness and her health.

"Stop for a minute," I told her, gently. "Look at what you experienced. It's not what a child should have gone through. It wasn't healthy. You're doing amazing considering where you came from." I saw a faint light dawning in Lisa's eyes, as if she'd let down her protective shields, just the tiniest bit.

The Canadian physician and renowned speaker and author Gabor Maté, MD, in his book *When the Body Says No*, discusses the importance of embracing "negative thinking." He defines negative thinking as a willingness to authentically inquire into the truth of what's happening. He writes, "When one lacks the capacity to feel heat, the risk of being burned increases."[31] He goes on to say, "Many people are blocked from self-knowledge and personal growth by the myth they feel compelled to hold on to, of having had a 'happy childhood.' A little negative thinking would empower them to see through the self-delusion that helps keep them stuck in self-harming behavioural patterns."[32]

The next time Lisa came to see me, she looked completely different. Her face and body had visibly relaxed and there was a new softness in her expression. "All this time I've just been thinking I'm a horrible adult," she said. "I was convinced my childhood had nothing to do with my struggles. Now I can see that my patterns are fear based—I was too afraid to let people in. I've been too afraid of rejection and had a lot of fears around intimacy and vulnerability. I saw all of that as weakness."

I felt an ache in my heart as Lisa continued, "Before, I simply yelled at myself internally and blamed myself for all the unhealthy things I was doing because it's my life and I'm obviously choosing these things. What I couldn't see was that this was my way to survive. No wonder this is my default mode, no wonder I always go here first. And I can feel how from this place, it will only take a gentle nudging to let this go because it isn't necessary anymore. I don't need to be angry at myself that I acted that way, but instead I can be appreciative that I found a way to survive. I can learn how to love it away instead of hating it and trying to cut it off."

Most of the clients who come to see me, like Lisa, have spent years trying different strategies and protocols in relation to their self-care—different diets, exercise plans, supplements, etc. And while they may have experienced short-term changes, nothing really stuck. And so often, like Lisa, they have internalized this pattern of failure, believing something is fundamentally wrong with them—for instance, that they are lazy and have no discipline. But it's clear something else is at work.

Imagine that you are swimming in an ocean with strong currents. You head out from the beach on a leisurely swim, intending just to move down the coastline a bit, and before you know it you look up and you have been pulled in the opposite direction and can no longer even see the beach that had been right there in front of you just a minute before. It can feel really scary and disorienting. The truth is that you can do all you want on the surface level—take swimming lessons to learn different strokes or build up your muscles to swim harder, but the reality is that you will still be swept away by the deeper currents underneath you. They will take you where they are going, regardless.

And so it is with your health journey. Until you come into a direct relationship with the deeper currents—seeing them, understanding them, and learning the source of their power—they will guide your journey without you having a say. You can try all the protocols you want, yet you will never be free to truly guide yourself toward your own thriving. Your shadows are those currents.

SHADOW AND SHAME

Where there is shame, there is shadow. Even if you are aware of what the shame is about on one level, there is something far deeper going on—the stories we have about ourselves, a trauma from the past, a cultural belief we've taken on. Oftentimes this boils down to some version of "there is something wrong with me." This is the territory of shame and it is sadly an intimate part of most of our journeys with self-care.

INQUIRY QUESTIONS

Let's bring this directly to your own experience now. One of the ways to uncover shadow is to use the shame you feel as an entry point. Now would be a great time to grab your journal and explore the following questions. Please remember that the degree of shadow that swirls with our shame can sometimes keep us so protected that we aren't able to access the really important, helpful part at the center of everything. Try sitting with yourself as you softly and gently explore these questions with an open curiosity and a willingness to be with your truth, whatever that may be.

+ What are the areas of the most shame for you on your health and self-care journey? In your life?

+ How does it feel now to name them? Have you shared them with anyone before? How did that feel?

+ What is most uncomfortable for you about these aspects of yourself? What feels most embarrassing? What feels most vulnerable?

+ What's your sense of what is underneath the shame? What feeds the shame?

+ How does the shame affect your level of motivation to create change?

+ What do you think might free you from the shame?

+ When you check in with yourself now, can you sense anything else that might be unacknowledged on the periphery? Perhaps it is something so central to what's going on for you that you haven't seen it?

What I've seen for many of us on our health journeys is that the combination of shadow and shame can trap us in a self-reinforcing cycle. First there are shadows at play, currents we can't see that are pulling us in this direction then that direction and preventing us from actualizing the changes that we seek. This is followed by the shame we then feel about where we've ended up as a result of these shadow currents, reinforcing patterns of self-sabotage and avoidance. Because of the shame, we repress the issues even further. We then create stories about ourselves, based on these layers of shame, remorse, and powerlessness, that explain, inaccurately, why we are not sustaining the changes we seek. By doing this we weigh ourselves down even more, allowing ourselves to be drawn even deeper into the shadow currents—making it that much harder to try to swim in the direction of thriving that we actually want to go. There's a sense of no escape.

In other words, the way in which we relate to ourselves on our journey of self-care is absolutely at the center of our capacity to create the changes we seek. And the way in which we relate to ourselves is intimately linked to how consciously we've explored the shadows at play.

CHECKING IN: *Pause for a moment and focus on your physical body; notice how all that you have been reading, absorbing, writing about, is touching and affecting you. What emotions are arising? What memories, images, or experiences are coming into your awareness as a result of the content of this chapter? Give yourself full permission to feel it all, to take your time, and to stay with your personal experiences as you continue to read.*

Have you ever had the experience of becoming upset about something that happened—perhaps you did something that felt embarrassing or that you regret—and then you spent days or weeks replaying the scenario in your mind, perhaps losing sleep over it? Finally, you reach out to a close friend or a counselor and share what happened. You cry. You admit to all the things that you are ashamed of or that upset you. You feel seen and heard. And most of all you feel loved and accepted.

Somehow, in being listened to in that way, with caring and loving attention, and sharing your truth, no matter how uncomfortable or embarrassing it might be, you feel lighter. The intensity of what you were carrying and grappling with for all that time dissipates. And your perspective shifts. What had felt so important and all-consuming no longer does. You have moved on and in the process feel more relaxed, whole, and accepting of yourself. This is what facing and embracing your shadows looks and feels like.

After Lisa first faced her shadows with me, she continued to open herself up in ways she could never have imagined. When I saw her some months later, she told me, "My capacity for feeling my emotions is really, really different—even in loving my children, which I always thought I did really well. When I was so busy numbing myself I didn't see the little twinkle behind my daughter's eye, or the little sadness. It's the subtleties that I notice now. When I am really present with someone, the connection is incredible. To choose not to be present is becoming more difficult for me. I think that when I see people now, I really *see* them. I'm relaxed being in my body and being present with that person in the moment. I just feel so much more than I felt before. I feel really alive."

Her health was shifting, too, now that she wasn't self-sabotaging. "I joined an Overeaters Anonymous group!" she added proudly. "I'm out there, connecting and sharing myself and being vulnerable. It feels amazing."

I'd like to return now to the analogy I shared in Key #1: the Mama Bear. What I love about the idea of mothering yourself in this way is that it weaves together the energy of deep compassion, unconditional love, and fierce, unwavering loyalty into one nurturing fabric.

It can seem like a contradiction to be fierce and courageous while also being gentle and loving. I've seen many folks (including myself when I first began engaging with shadow work) get into an orientation of needing to "root out" all the bad stuff. There can be a belief that shadow work is about purifying and removing what is wrong with you. And it is certainly understandable how our minds could create such an idea—after all, there's a reason that we've shoved these parts of ourselves into the unconscious dark corners. It's scary territory!

Yet shadow work is quite the opposite. It's the compassion and self-acceptance of your inner Mama Bear that will lead you down the pathway to your inner freedom. The courageous fierceness keeps you in the process even when it is really hard. The compassion and unconditional love allow you to accept and embrace those parts of yourself that may seem ugly, wrong, horrible, or too much. Shadow work means having the courage to take off the masks—the habitual ways in which you pretend to be someone else or hide your truth. And you may not even be conscious you are wearing them until you begin opening into this work.

Here's the real kicker: as Jung said, it's not all "bad" stuff. Facing and embracing your shadows also means choosing to own who you uniquely are, to reveal your particular genius, to allow your gifts to shine out into the world. This is sometimes referred to as the "golden shadow." And from what I've seen in my clients and myself, this territory can be the cause of so many self-limiting and addictive behaviors—stronger even than the "dark" shadows. We're so afraid of our greatness!

The shadow healing work that I've engaged with has allowed my life-energy to blossom and bloom. It's helped me to feel more naturally comfortable being fully "me" on all levels. I've seen a direct relationship with my capacity to see and own my gifts and the courage to continually step through fears and doubts so that I can offer those gifts to the world. From my own experience, I can intimately say that being in a direct, honest relationship with your fears, doubts, and insecurities is the doorway to birthing and offering your true self to the world, and giving yourself permission to shine! This may be for you (as it was for me) one of the most terrifying aspects of facing and embracing your shadows, of owning ALL of who you are.

INQUIRY QUESTIONS

Let's pause here for a moment and give you a chance to explore this for yourself. You can grab your journal if you like and see what shows up for you in the following questions:

+ Where might you have a "golden shadow" at play, keeping your light dimmed, your true self boxed up? How and when do you hide your gifts, or avoid letting yourself be seen?

+ What are you afraid might be revealed if you allowed yourself to thrive? What might you be afraid of losing? Do you have fears about how your thriving might affect the people around you?

The author and integrative-medicine pioneer Rachel Naomi Remen writes the following: "Reclaiming ourselves usually means coming to recognize and accept that we have in us both sides of everything. We are capable of fear and courage, generosity and selfishness, vulnerability and strength.

These things do not cancel each other out but offer us a full range of power and response to life. Life is as complex as we are."[33]

Each time I've engaged with shadow work, I've come away feeling freer, lighter, and more at home in myself. My life-energy is less and less bound up in protecting and hiding from my truth. As I embrace the disowned parts of myself, consciously integrating them, it is like I am no longer leaking energy. As a result, my chronic fatigue has gradually dissipated.

It takes a lot of your life-energy to protect, hide, and pretend to be something you're not, whether you are conscious of that or not. The disowned parts of yourself are like holes in your life vessel, draining your life-energy away. Although the part of the boat that is above the water looks intact, the hull is punctured and the keel is broken, so you're being blown around, unable to steer a course that's in alignment with truth. Other people may not be able to see it, but you're taking in more water than you can bail out, and you're being helplessly carried by the deeper currents.

When we consciously shine light on the shadows, shedding and releasing all the layers of protection that we've built up around them, accepting all of who we are, it is like breaking out of prison. We free ourselves, and our life-energy.

Can you feel what would be possible if you were completely at home in yourself? So many of the pathologies playing out in ourselves and the world these days are because of the incessant *dis*-ease that we feel in our own bodies and our own lives. As author and speaker Byron Katie says, "I am a lover of what is, not because I'm a spiritual person, but because it hurts when I argue with reality."[34]

SHADOW DIPLOMACY

As Jung knew, there is no specific technique or proven tactic for dealing with the shadow. As he wrote, "There is, as a matter of fact, no technique at all. . . . It is rather a dealing comparable to diplomacy or statesmanship. . . . First of all, one has to accept and to take seriously into account the existence of the shadow. Secondly, it is necessary to be informed about its qualities and intentions. Thirdly, long and difficult negotiations will be unavoidable. . . . Nobody can know what the final outcome of such negotiations will be. One only knows that through careful collaboration the problem itself becomes changed."[35]

In this spirit of diplomacy, negotiation, and collaboration, one of the most powerful tools I've found for dealing with the shadow is the Voice Dialogue technique, created by clinical psychologists Hal and Sidra Stone, originators of the Psychology of Selves. Voice Dialogue is a therapeutic technique in which we get to play with the myriad of different perspectives within ourselves that we name as voices. Hal Stone describes it as "dialogue with the family of selves that lives within each of us."[36] In my work with clients I will often weave elements of Voice Dialogue into our engagement as a way to reveal and uncover aspects of the shadows.

When we're entrenched with our identification with certain voices in our heads, we see those voices as being "who we are." The loud voices—like the voice of shame and the voice of self-judgment—become "me." We believe that what those voices are saying is "truth." In a sense, we cage ourselves into a very small and limited conception of who we are. By using Voice Dialogue, we can loosen that identification and begin to discover the flexibility and capacity necessary to embody and understand different perspectives within ourselves. We can come to recognize that the inner voices that have caused us so much pain, voices that we've been identifying with, are actually only a few out of an infinitely wide spectrum of viewpoints inside of us. Through consciously playing with these different voices in ourselves, we can begin to strengthen some of the softer voices that have been bullied into silence and submission, in some cases for a lifetime. We can invite these voices into conversation with each other.

Sidra describes how when she and her husband Hal first stumbled upon the power of this practice, he asked her to move to another part of the room and become a vulnerable child rather than just talking about it:

I left the couch I'd been sitting on, sat on the floor next to the coffee table, put my head down on it and suddenly everything changed. I became absolutely quiet and experienced the world around me differently. Sounds, colors and feelings were more intense than before.

The sophisticated, rational, articulate woman with all the answers was gone and in her place was a very young child. I was extremely quiet and very sensitive to everything in my surroundings. I responded to energies rather than thoughts. I felt things I had not felt in decades, and knew things that were not known by my everyday mind. I knew, without question, the realities of my soul. After about an hour, Hal asked me to move to my original seat on the couch and I returned to my previous way of being in the world . . . but my little girl was still with me and I would never lose her completely again.[37]

While the Voice Dialogue technique is something that works best when guided by a skilled practitioner so that you have the outside reflection and witnessing that help to reveal the shadows, you can also explore it on your own.

Find a private, quiet space with your journal. You can explore the voices in a journal or speak them out loud. Both practices can be very powerful. Choose a voice—"the critic" for example—that you want to enter into dialogue with. Ask a question of your critic like, "How are you feeling?" or "What are your needs?" If you are doing this with a partner, he or she can ask the questions.

This is where you allow yourself to become that voice and respond from it. It can be helpful to make an obvious acknowledgment of some kind when you are shifting voices so that you can help your consciousness to fully embrace the different perspectives. Moving your body as you shift, walking to the other side of the room, swapping chairs, or changing the quality of your voice can help you to drop more fully into releasing your former perspective and embracing the new one.

Try to play around right now with this practice and see what happens. If you're journaling, you may want to leave aside the questioning and just allow stream-of-consciousness writing to flow out as that voice. You might get in touch with some of the different voices that live inside of you—perhaps a "shame" voice, the voice of "resistance," the "perfectionist," the "skeptic." Or you might even get clearer and more specific and recognize the voice of your biological father or mother that has gotten trapped in your own head. Ask the different voices questions to find out what their perspectives have to say. If you continue to explore, you will probably discover a validity and truth in each of the voices, even in the hardest ones to hear. There is no "right" and "wrong" here—just a multiplicity of perspectives. This is where the tender vulnerability comes in, and the necessity for gentle, loving care on this journey.

Once you begin to name some of the habitual voices inside you, to get a feel for their tone and unique personalities and opinions, then you can get playful and begin to invite in voices of your choosing to see what they have to say. I like to think of the practice of Voice Dialogue as inviting more voices to the table. The habitual ones are already gathered at the table, so you can invite more, less-dominant voices to join the conversation. Sometimes the new voices you invite might be very quiet at first; perhaps they have never spoken before inside of you in a way that you could hear them.

I introduced Lisa to this practice, and she found it tremendously liberating. "I always thought that the harsh, critical voice in my head was like the judge and jury—it had the truth and the final answer. Now, I've learned to laugh and relax with what I hear in my head. I can hear echoes of my father in that voice, and I can tell it, 'Okay, I've heard you, now does anybody else have anything to say?' I discovered that there were other voices inside, like the nurturer, my inner mother, the gardener. The loudest voice that I typically heard wasn't necessarily the truth for me."

INQUIRY QUESTIONS

Now that you have gotten a feel for how Voice Dialogue works, grab your journal and explore more fully which voices are already at the table, and which ones you might like to invite in:

- ✦ What are the loud habitual voices at the table for you (e.g., the voice of resistance, the critic, self-judger, perfectionist, rebel)?

- ✦ What are others voices you might invite to join (e.g., the nurturer, the wise grandmother, your loyal friend, your inner rockstar!)? Let your creativity go wild here.

- ✦ What different kinds of perspectives and guidance can you imagine opening to if the table got rounded out with more voices?

- ✦ What are some more voices that have your back, that are focused on guiding you toward your own thriving?

- ✦ How might you align yourself more fully with those voices, while also not denying the other voices at the table?

By turning toward what we have not wanted to face, we free ourselves from prisons we didn't even realize we were in. By revealing our fears, insecurities, and self-judgments, by embracing our shame, and by being completely honest with ourselves, we liberate ourselves. Even the kindest, most gentle, and loving voices can be deep in the shadows. Each time we invite other voices to the table, inviting in perspectives that have not been up to now a part of our inner sense of self, we free up more of our true self to come through. From doing this practice, I personally have experienced physical effects—I can breathe more fully, and my body somehow feels more substantial.

As we come to the close of this key, I want to emphasize again that with shadows *we can't see what we can't see.* Shadow work can thus be hard to do alone. We may need others to help shine light on what we've been blind to and to help us to hold ourselves with greater compassion and understanding. I have no doubt whatsoever of the vital importance of inviting others into our healing journey (I've devoted Key #8: Inviting Support and Connection to the topic because it is absolutely essential).

Facing and embracing your shadows is a gradual ongoing process. It helps us clear away the clutter on a regular basis, to keep ourselves as clear, bright, free, and alive as we can be. As you learn to more compassionately embrace your complexity and your wholeness, this second key, Facing and Embracing Your Shadows, will open the doorway for you to rest and relax more easily into all of who you are, without apology and without hiding. This is absolutely foundational in order to embody and live in true health. You cannot thrive if you are not at ease. You cannot thrive if you are not able to embrace, accept, and relax into your wholeness.

We humans are complex, paradoxical, mysterious, and flawed. All of us. And therein lies our beauty. As Lisa now lovingly says of herself, "I'm a beautiful, worthwhile mess in progress." This isn't a quick fix, but an ongoing process. You can't just check this off your list and be done. As you explore, I again encourage you to do so with your fierce Mama Bear energy—with gentleness, love, and nourishing care for yourself. In welcoming and embracing all of who you are, your shadows and your light, you come home to yourself. You blossom. Your unique life expression is able to shine out into the world.

KEY #3

STRENGTHENING YOUR SELF-AWARENESS MUSCLES

*"Not biology, but ignorance of ourselves,
has been the key to our powerlessness."*
—ADRIENNE RICH

I'M SURE YOU'VE come across headlines like this one when browsing the news over your morning coffee: STUDIES SHOW THAT A LOW-CARB, HIGH-FAT DIET IMPROVES WEIGHT LOSS. And perhaps you've thought, *Wait a minute. I thought everyone was still talking about how fat was supposed to be bad?* A few clicks of your mouse and, sure enough, you will find a whole host of respectable-looking studies that appear to directly contradict the headline you just read. And so it goes on. PALEO DIET MELTS AWAY FAT! PALEO DIET LINKED TO RISING OBESITY. COFFEE INCREASES RISK OF HEART ATTACKS. COFFEE LINKED TO GREATER LONGEVITY. Oh, and apparently, BONE BROTH IS THE NEW COFFEE. MAMMOGRAMS SAVE LIVES. MAMMOGRAMS LINKED TO HIGHER CANCER RISKS. For every study about some particular approach to diet or health, it seems, a contradictory one can be found. And in the Internet Age, they're all just a click away. From one week to the next new fads emerge, and each is held up as being the latest, greatest answer to all our ills—until the next one comes along.

The good news is we've never been more empowered to be partners in our own healthcare, armed with the infinite knowledge that Google can provide. Gone are the days when we had to take the doctor's words as gospel because, to be honest, we didn't even understand what half those words meant. Now, we can do our own research, figure out our options, and make informed decisions—at least, in theory. The bad news is, it's up to us to navigate between the endless, conflicting messages we will find, many of which seem quite legitimate. And everyone we speak to seems to consider themselves a health expert—our friends, our colleagues, our mothers, our therapists, our hair-stylists, our neighbors, and on it goes. Many of the clients who come to me feel overwhelmed by information and opinions but are lacking the capacity to discriminate and sift through it all.

What I also notice, with many of these people, is that while they're listening to everyone around them, they're not listening to the most important source of information and wisdom about their health: their own body. And when I say body, I'm not just referring to the physical body, but to all dimensions of who you are—physical, mental, emotional, and spiritual— that are housed in your unique body-home. Key #3: Strengthening Your Self-Awareness Muscles opens the door to a new kind of empowerment by showing you how to tune in to the feedback your body-home is giving you. Until you cultivate your self-awareness, you won't be able to truly take authorship of your life. If you are unconscious of your body's feedback, the only things guiding your choices are external messages—from "experts," health fads, and friends, to the latest studies.

BECOMING YOUR OWN HEALTH GUIDE

When we only get our health information externally, we end up taking care of ourselves in a way that reminds me of using an IKEA manual—following a guide that someone else put together to create a predesigned product. And yet you are not a piece of furniture that comes with a standardized set of tools, a finite number of pieces, and only one simple method of assembly. No one can write a manual for you—you are far too complex and nuanced. You are much more like a craftsman-made piece of furniture. You couldn't even write a manual for yourself, as there is nothing static about you. You are an alive, evolving, dynamic being, and you are utterly unique.

So many things have shaped, and continue to shape, the particular human being you are in this very moment: your genetics; the cultures and environments in which you've been planted; the particular mosaic of traumas and challenges you've experienced and faced, and how you adapted and coped with them; what behavioral patterns have been modeled for you; how you choose to eat, exercise, and so on. You have your own constitutional tendencies, too. Do you tend to run cold or hot? Do you typically feel dry or moist? Do you find yourself to be really grounded or do you float effortlessly from thing to thing? Your preferences, how your body responds to stimuli, the areas in which you are weaker and stronger, what lights you up and brings you alive—these are all born from the complex interweaving of all of the influences on you before you are born and throughout your lifetime. You resonate, relate, and interact with the world in your own specific way. No matter how much science progresses and can tell us incredible things about how the human body works and what supports it, the end result can never negate your uniqueness. You are too complex to be boiled down to a set of protocols and rules.

Of course, you do have fundamental needs that you share with all other humans. Just as you need to tend to your plants by providing water, nutrients, and sunlight to help them grow and thrive, you need to tend to your basic needs. Yet there are many ways to nourish yourself, to tend to those needs. You might absolutely love playing tennis, while your friend Janet would much rather go swimming, as she finds tennis places too much strain on her body. And no matter how healthy spinach is supposed to be for you, perhaps you simply can't stand it! You would rather eat kale every day. Clearly, we can learn from the abundance of experts out there who are writing books, who have transformed their own lives with certain approaches and methods, but no set of healthy habits will ever be sustainable until you make them your own.

No one else but you can feel, sense, and know the various impacts of what you are engaging with, what you are taking into your body, how it feels to be working at your job, what's happening for you in your relationships. You are the only one with direct access to that information. If you rely on someone else to tell you what you need to be doing to be healthy, you're discounting the fact that no one else can actually do that for you. No one but you can feel the impact of your choices on your vitality. No one else has the capacity to have that perspective and empowered clarity. It doesn't matter how many years they have been in school or what letters they have after their names, they can never ever know what it feels like for YOU.

If you can't rely on a set of rules and guidelines someone else has come up with, then how do you take care of yourself in a way that truly honors you? That's where strengthening your self-awareness comes in. You need to learn how to receive and heed the feedback that is continuously coming from your body-home. You have the opportunity to become an expert in your own health—not a health expert in general, but an expert in *your* health. And it starts by simply paying attention. Ask yourself, for example, How do you feel after you eat a particular food? What time of day do you feel most energetic? What types of exercise do you enjoy? How does being at work affect your mood?

LISTEN TO YOUR BODY

You alone can choose to become deeply intimate, attuned, and sensitive to what your life-energy is sharing with you all the time. You have the opportunity to live in direct relationship with yourself, to consciously look through your eyes, feel through your senses, and know your unique ways of perceiving your particular life experiences. Strengthening your self-awareness opens you up to understanding and honoring your uniqueness, and learning what truly nourishes you on all levels.

In our technology-rich age, there are many tools and methods available that can help you to listen to, and learn more about, your body. The term "quantified self," for example, refers to the growing movement of using technology to gather data and statistics, or "biometrics," about your own body. One of the most common biometric tools is the wearable "activity monitor," like a Fitbit, that will track your activity levels throughout the day. There are also devices that will measure your food consumption, the quality of the air you breathe, the quality of your sleep, your blood-oxygen or hormone levels, your fertility cycles, and so on, with new gadgets and smartphone apps being created every day. You can also go even further and get your own DNA sequenced, to better be able to predict genetic predispositions and risks.

These tools can be useful, to a point, and I'll be returning to some of them in the next chapter when we discuss how you can learn to regulate yourself. However, as you begin to engage with self-awareness, I'd encourage you to primarily focus on receiving feedback directly from your body, without the technological middleman. The danger with these technologies is that if you haven't developed your capacity to listen to your body from the inside, so to speak, they become yet another form of external "expert."

If you become reliant on them to know what's happening inside, you will actually reduce your capacity for direct listening. So while I leave it up to you to decide whether you want to integrate these kinds of technologies into your self-awareness journey, I'd caution you to do so only in close conjunction with the practices of paying attention that I'll be teaching in this chapter.

Now, if you are like most of the people I know (including myself!), paying attention to your own body is not something that comes naturally, not a skill you were taught as a kid. I spent most of my childhood with a stuffy nose. For eleven years I was given allergy shots that didn't seem to do much of anything. It was only as an adult, through the awareness that I developed on my healing journey, that I discovered that I was sensitive to dairy, a prime culprit for childhood congestion.

Even those of us who have developed powerful self-awareness in other areas of life too often stop short of applying it to our health. In my journey, I have encountered many adults who have consciously developed their self-awareness in profound ways through spiritual growth, through learning in relationships, through traumatic experiences, and through therapy. But no matter how clearly we see in some domains, we can still be blind in others. And as I discussed in Key #2: Facing and Embracing Your Shadows, we can't see what we are blind to.

Most adults are largely illiterate when it comes to being able to read the feedback signals we are receiving all the time from our bodies. We simply haven't learned the language. For most of us, it feels foreign to drop into our bodies and listen, feel, and ask for what we need. So we interpret the signals in ways that fit into the languages we know. For instance, Jane, a friend with chronic insomnia, drinks a few cups of coffee a day to deal with her exhaustion, not realizing that she is sensitive to caffeine and her insomnia is largely due to that. Her body, through its exhaustion, is trying to let her know that she needs to rest, relax, and support herself in getting restorative sleep. Her insomnia is letting her know that something is causing her nervous system to be in an excited "fight-or-flight" response (in this case, the caffeine could be the prime culprit).

Paul, another friend, suffers from persistent headaches for which he takes painkillers, declaring that he doesn't have any choice—he needs to go to work and keep his company afloat. By numbing out the pain, he's also numbing out his body's message that his job stress is not healthy. These are simple, yet all too common, examples that I hope will help you begin learning the language of your own body.

Often the language of our body's feedback is quite simple, but it is made more complex by what's happening in our shadows (hence the importance of Key #2) and by the strength of cultural norms and beliefs. For Jane, the simple message is that she is receiving the feedback that she is exhausted, and therefore she should prioritize rest and sleep in order to renew herself. This seems to be one of the hardest things for folks to do in our culture, and Jane is no exception. As a child she was scolded for being fat and lazy, and the shadow issues she has created around this are obscuring the voice of her exhausted body. I can't tell you how many people, like Jane, come to me with a primary complaint of fatigue or a sense of nearing burnout, and my main work is helping them to find a way of allowing themselves to rest. With so many commitments, the cultural belief that we ought to be going strong on six hours of sleep, and our life-energy invested in things that don't actually energize us, it's no wonder we're exhausted.

Sometimes, jumping too quickly—or taking a shortcut—to seek relief from our symptoms will cut us off from the messages, like Paul taking pain-killers. One of my clients, Christy, noticed a pattern she had around emotional eating. Home after a stressful, hectic day at work, she would reach for the Ben & Jerry's. After we'd been working together for a while, she decided to experiment with not reaching for the ice cream. When she felt the urge, instead of heading for the freezer, she asked herself: What do I really want? What does my body really need? Is it that bowl full of sugar and fat, or is that simply standing in for something else? And does it actually fill the void? How does it make me feel? She became aware that after eating the ice cream, she usually felt dull and lacking in energy. Her body was telling her that she craved something—but perhaps that something was actually love, or comfort, or connection. She decided to drink some fresh water and take a beautiful walk with her husband, and she came back feeling revitalized and refreshed.

What I've seen repeatedly with my clients is that once I help them to begin to mother themselves in a loving, nurturing way (Key #1), break through some of the shadow currents and cultural beliefs that aren't serving them (Key #2), and cultivate an awareness of and trust in the wisdom and guidance they are receiving from their body-home (Key #3), then they are well on their way to feeling empowered and skillful in guiding themselves toward their most thriving self.

At this point, I'm not asking you to do anything particular with the information you receive. This third key is simply about developing greater awareness, while Key #4: Cultivating Resilience will help you begin to respond and adapt to the messages you receive and start to positively impact your health. You can only change what you can perceive, so don't skip too quickly over the awareness. Here is a simple meditative inquiry you can use to start to get in touch with your own body and embody this key by strengthening your self-awareness muscles.

🎧 SELF-AWARENESS MEDITATION: *As we begin, see if you can let down and let go of whatever it is you've been holding today. Feel yourself relax into where you are sitting or lying right now, allowing the weight of your body to really sink in and be held by gravity. Invite the whole of your awareness to come home into your body and your being in this moment. Bring your conscious awareness into your body as if it is your first time, feeling the intense curiosity that comes with that: What does it feel like to be alive and in a body?*

As a conscious curious explorer of yourself, allow your awareness to tune into how it feels to be breathing right now. Can you notice the subtleties of the air flowing in and out, of your diaphragm dropping down to allow your lungs to expand and invite air in? And can you feel the beat of your heart and the pulsation of the blood moving through your entire body, out to the ends of your limbs, up into your brain, feeding all the organ systems? Can you sense your life-energy in this moment? Can you feel yourself in relationship with the environment that you're in? Can you feel and acknowledge whatever your emotional space or state might be in this moment? Can you scan your day (or yesterday), feeling a bodily connection with the different choices you've made—the things you've eaten, the places you've been, the people you've interacted with, the ways you've moved your body? Can you identify the moments when you've felt most alive, clear, and connected in the last twenty-four hours? Are you aware of when you have felt the most depleted?

See if you can flip through your recent history, and perhaps even some of your more distant history, much as you would flip through a book, to get little tastes and memories of the ways in which you have guided yourself to arrive where you are right now.

Can you identify the perspectives or priorities that have been shaping the choices you've been making? Can you feel how you've been turning toward or turning away from yourself? Who or what have been served by your choices? What sacrifices might you be making? Can you identify some competing commitments, that sense of having different priorities that might seem at odds with each other? What are those different priorities, and do you have a sense of which ones tend to win out over the others habitually?

In the above meditation, you explored what it is to expand your sense of intimacy and awareness of yourself. From this little taste, can you get a sense of the possibilities of how you can deepen in your felt knowing of how the various choices you are making are affecting you—physically, mentally, emotionally, and spiritually?

This process is like gathering data from all of your different ways of sensing and knowing. This includes your physical senses, your intuition, your emotional feedback, the state of your thoughts, the behavioral choices you make, and how connected you feel with the deepest, most essential aspects of what it is to be alive.

It also includes taking note of not just what you are taking into your body, but what you are releasing as well. Yes, that means your poop and a whole lot more! Culturally, many of us have been taught to have an aversion to that sort of thing. Yet can you see the potential here for yourself? If you are truly your own best health guide, then consider yourself the first doctor you go to, before you seek out any other opinions or perspectives. So wouldn't you want to train yourself to be as familiar as you can with the data your body is sharing with you? As a conscious curious explorer of yourself, this is all you have to do: simply gather the data, then observe the patterns and what it is they are trying to tell you. All the data is indeed guiding you, every moment of your life.

This is preventative healthcare at its best. When you cultivate this level of intimacy with yourself, you can begin to fine-tune the choices you are making in subtler and subtler ways. It's not just about food and exercise. Every single choice you make throughout your day influences the state of your vitality. Wouldn't you like to be making informed choices based on your own self-knowing?

Here's the thing: The feedback can start off very soft and gentle, like a friendly whisper in your ear. Yet if you don't seem to be hearing it (perhaps because you haven't yet cultivated the ability to do so, or because you are

KEY #3: STRENGTHENING YOUR SELF-AWARENESS MUSCLES   73

simply ignoring it), the feedback gets louder, and Louder, and LOUDER, until it can feel like you ran into a brick wall at full speed. This is what it felt like for me when I collapsed into my deep fatigue in my mid-twenties. Looking back, I can see that the feedback, the data, had been there for a long time. I just didn't know how to consciously receive it. I hadn't learned the language. This key, Strengthening Your Self-Awareness Muscles, allows you to build your capacity to hear the feedback when it is a soft and loving nudge, rather than the forceful smack over the head.

Strengthening your self-awareness is a lifelong process. As the great sage J. Krishnamurti wrote, "I am learning about myself from moment to moment, and the 'myself' is extraordinarily vital; it is living, moving, it has no beginning and no end. When I say, 'I know myself', learning has come to an end in accumulated knowledge. Learning is never cumulative; it is a movement of knowing which has no beginning and no end."[38]

This awareness practice doesn't always require effort and vigilance. Recently I was looking for a new winter coat, and I noticed that after doing some research online about what I might want, my attention naturally became attuned to outerwear. Everywhere I went, my eyes were drawn to coats that women were wearing. I had never really noticed them before—the features, the colors, the brands, the styles—but now that I wanted one for myself, my awareness had been switched on.

Strengthening your self-awareness muscles in relation to your health works in the same way. You'll discover that once you begin to bring conscious attention to something, all of a sudden it is in your face all the time. My clients will often report how incredibly uncomfortable that can feel. They are no longer blind or numb to their patterns around eating, sleeping, addictive tendencies, etc. There can be a period of hyperawareness where it can almost feel like getting slapped in the face constantly with things that had just been part of your ways of being.

I typically suggest that clients hang out in this stage for a while (even though sometimes it can be uncomfortable). It gives you a relaxed time to simply observe yourself, the patterns, the influences, and the subtleties and nuances of what is happening, without any pressure to change anything. This is crucial! In the kinds of cultural contexts that most of us find ourselves in these days, we can easily apply a sense of urgency and pressure to jump into action and immediately create the changes we seek.

In taking spacious time to become intimately aware of what's happening for you, you'll find that when you are ready to move into creating conscious change in behavior or thought or life circumstance, your choices are rooted in an abundance of data and context. Therefore, you will be able to create a strategy that is uniquely suited for you. Your capacity to observe what happens with the change will empower you in this ongoing guidance of yourself. We'll explore this possibility more in the next key. But first, give yourself as much time as you need to simply pay attention and become deeply intimate with what is going on.

Staying with this discomfort and loving yourself through all of it requires many of the things we've learned in the first two keys—the courageous, fierce love of your inner Mama Bear and the vulnerability to shine a light on your shadows.

CHECKING IN: *Take a deep breath and check in with how you are feeling right now. What is all of this evoking for you? How can you hold yourself gently and lovingly as you open into this new territory?*

TAKING STOCK OF YOUR VITALITY AND HEALTH

To begin exercising your self-awareness muscles, and in the spirit of the deep listening that I've been describing in this chapter, here are some suggested areas of life you might pay attention to. Start with those areas where you feel like you struggle most in relation to your self-care: Diet? Sleep? Having downtime? Exercise? Relationships? Work? From the list below, choose the areas that feel the most relevant to present-day you. Then consider what kinds of data and feedback you would like to receive.

DIGESTION, NUTRITION, & EATING: Ah, the complicated topic of food. While you've probably already gathered that I am not a fan of the myriad of fad diets and changing theories that spin us around and around, I am a fan of empowerment. Understanding your digestive system, how it works, and what you can do to support its optimal functioning has been, in my experience on my own health journey and the health journeys of my clients, foundational to vitality. Developing an attentive, conscious relationship with your eating patterns impacts how you receive and digest the foods that you eat.

Notice what foods you are drawn to and what foods repel you. Notice how you feel when you're eating them, how present you are as you eat, and how that affects the way you feel afterward. As you eat, do you feel connected to where your food comes from? How does your mood influence your enjoyment of your food as well as how you digest? Pay attention to whether there is a connection between the foods you eat and any intolerance or allergic reactions. You might ask yourself the following questions: What foods are comforting to me? What foods seem to make me come alive? What foods make me feel tired and deadened?

How your body responds to the foods you are eating is not just about the breakdown of the nutrients. You respond uniquely and might find that certain foods make you feel tired or depressed, or give you gas, or make you feel especially nourished. And how you are feeling emotionally as you eat also greatly impacts the quality of your digestion. If you are distracted by something very stressful going on in your life or are busy at work and hardly even notice the food going in your mouth, that impacts the ways in which your body will assimilate what you are taking in.

One practice I often suggest to support clients in becoming more intimate with their patterns around eating, food, and its impacts is the experiment of keeping a diet diary for a few days. Now, this isn't the kind of diet diary that often comes with weight-loss diets. The point of it is to expand your awareness of yourself, not to count calories. The categories I suggest for a comprehensive diet diary are as follows: date; time; foods eaten (including drinks, supplements, and medications); feelings (emotions, stress levels); bowel and urine patterns; gas; main activities (such as working on the computer, exercise, cleaning the house, commuting, playing with the kids, business meetings).

YOUR BREATH: Breathing is one of the most fundamental human activities, and yet most of us never give it a second's thought. Of course, from one perspective that's a good thing—if we had to remember to breathe, we might be in trouble! But most of us were never taught to breathe in a way that is optimal. We breathe how we breathe and that's it. Yet your breath is an incredible, empowering doorway to influence so much of your body's physiology, your mental/emotional states, and your sense of spiritual connection, as I'll be sharing in the next key. For now, I'd like to invite you into a breath inquiry. Notice how you are breathing at this very moment. What parts of you move as you breathe in, and as you breathe out? Would you describe your breath as fast or slow? Deep or shallow? Would you describe your breath cycle as smooth or does it include gaps? As you bring this awareness into your daily life, take note of how your breath changes throughout your day in response to different situations and/or emotions. And if you play around with the pace and depth of your breath, how does that affect how you are feeling?

YOUR THOUGHTS & EMOTIONS: When you start paying attention to what's going on emotionally and physically as you move through your day, you will see that your thoughts and emotions have big physiological impacts on your body at every moment. If you are feeling stressed emotionally about something at work or in a relationship, it will be mirrored in your body. Some of these changes may be happening at a level you are not conscious of, but as you develop your self-awareness, you will start to notice certain patterns.

As you are moving through your life, try to bring greater awareness to how your thoughts and emotions are landing in your body, becoming present to the various dimensions of the feelings and sensations. With practice you may start to be able to track and sequence them throughout your body. See if you can notice how your posture, facial expressions, and the other ways you hold your body influence your perspectives and outlook. Consciously shift how you are being in your body and see what happens. When you feel yourself in a stress reaction, practice bringing awareness to the sensations in the body—your heart rate, breath quality and rate, perspiration, the temperature of your hands and feet, salivation, muscle tension, etc. By shifting your attitude to one of curiosity, your state of being may begin to shift toward greater relaxation without you actively trying to do so. Try it and see what happens.

YOUR SLEEP: See if you can pay attention to the quality of your sleep and to how you feel when you wake up in the morning. Are you feeling rested? If you know you haven't gotten enough sleep, think back to the choices you made and the activities you engaged in during the day. Is there a connection? Take note of any stimulating substances you've used, such as caffeinated beverages, medications, herbs, or supplements. Note when you have used them and the quantity. Likewise take note of any relaxing substances you took into your body, again noting how much and when you used them. What is your current sleep environment like? What are your current evening and bedtime routines? How do they support or not support you in dropping into a restful, rejuvenating sleep? What time do you go to bed? What time do you wake up? What is the average amount of sleep you get each night? Does that feel optimal for you? How does having non-optimal sleep affect you throughout the day that follows? You might try keeping a diary for a week to get a clearer picture of your patterns around sleep. You can use the above questions as a guideline of the kinds of things to note for yourself.

RELAXATION & PLAY: How often do you take time to truly relax and just have fun? For some of us as adults, it may feel like we need to learn again how to truly let down and play in a way that deeply renews us (something we'll return to in Key #6). Physiologically, so much happens in our nervous system and our body's biochemistry that gives us ample feedback about the undeniable impact that rest and play have on our health and vitality. Pay attention to how you feel when you give yourself the gift of unstructured time that is purely for your enjoyment. Notice how much difference the simplest things can make—a shared laugh with a good friend, sitting for a few minutes in the sunshine, playing with your dog, your cat, or your child. Notice if you have a resistance to the idea of play: Are there shadow issues that might be preventing you from allowing yourself this restorative time? If you find yourself feeling drained and reaching for the coffee, experiment with taking a short walk somewhere beautiful instead, and see which rejuvenates you more.

MOVEMENT & FLEXIBILITY: Notice how your body responds to the different movements you ask it to perform—from simple everyday things like climbing stairs or walking to the grocery store, to more complex movements required by various forms of sport or exercise. Notice how flexible your body is: What activities come naturally and what feel hard or even impossible to do? What forms of movement do you enjoy, and what activities are unpleasant or feel unnatural for you? Pay attention to the postures you find yourself in at work, whether you are standing for long hours, sitting behind a computer, or doing something physically demanding. How does your body respond?

SEXUALITY: It is amazing to me how something so fundamental to our vitality is largely neglected in health conversations or talked about in shadowy, indirect ways. Your sexual energy is your life-energy, your innate creative force. You can connect with, move, and explore your sexual energy regardless of whether you are by yourself or in intimate play with another person. How are you opening to experience sensual and sexual pleasure these days? Pay attention to this area of your life: Does it feel vital, satisfying, and alive, or is it something you avoid or feel frustrated about? How at ease do you feel in your sexuality? Is it uncomfortable territory for you? If you engage in sexual activity with yourself or a partner, notice how you feel before, during, and after.

ATTENTION: We live in a time when our attention seems destined to be divided and fragmented much of the time. We've become accustomed to multitasking—keeping one eye on our emails while we're having a conversation on the phone, checking Facebook while putting the kids to bed, watching TV while we exercise at the gym. Notice your attention habits, particularly in relationship to technology. Pay attention to how you feel when you're trying to do three things at once. What happens if you leave your phone aside for an hour? Can you focus all of your attention on another person when needed? What comes up for you if you sit quietly with yourself for fifteen minutes? What do you experience when you spend time in nature?

ELIMINATION PATHWAYS: Sadly, the nourishment of our elimination pathways is often neglected on our health journeys. We may concentrate more on what we're taking in, but not think as much about how we can support, on an ongoing basis, the release of what we no longer need. Strengthening your awareness of your elimination pathways is about taking note of the quality, odor, appearance, and quantities of what your body is releasing all the time. Yes, this is a dignified way of talking about your poop, your pee, your sweat, and your breath. These are the ways your body lets go of what it no longer needs, and they can tell you a whole lot about how your body is functioning, how it is liking (or not liking) what you are taking in, and what you might be able to do to better support yourself.

How often do you sweat profusely? What about even sweating a little bit? How much water are you typically drinking each day? What circumstances increase the amount, or decrease the amount? How often do you pee on a daily basis? And what is its color? What is the odor of your breath? Does it change at various times of the day? How often do you poop each day? What is the odor and appearance of it? How do the foods you eat influence that? These are just some examples of the areas around which you can grow your awareness of your physical elimination pathways.

Elimination is not just limited to the physical organ systems, however. We all need to move through and release strong thoughts and emotions as well, otherwise they can morph into physical tension or get somaticized into various kinds of illness. Are there ways that you currently support the movement and release of these subtler aspects of yourself?

As you can probably tell from what I've shared thus far, strengthening your self-awareness muscles takes time and practice. Yet the difference here is that *you are consciously cultivating the foundation for a lifelong journey.* This is not a quick fix. As leadership coach Robbie Gass states, "Like an ability or a muscle, hearing your inner wisdom is strengthened by doing it."[39] This is about engaging in a master's level study of yourself so that you can feel empowered, confident, strong, clear, and trusting in your capacity to guide yourself toward your own thriving. You are here to support yourself to be the most alive, vibrant version of you that you can be!

If you're feeling overwhelmed by the complexity that is you, don't worry. Being your own number one health guide doesn't mean being your *only* health guide. But through the application of this key you will be able to engage with all the other authorities—starting with your doctors and health practitioners—while being in charge of your own health journey. As you own your own expertise, you can seek out the professionals and support you need in a way that serves you best. You can ask the questions that you need to ask. You can receive guidance and filter that guidance through your own self-knowing. You can have discernment about whom you want to have on your team of support (something we'll talk more about in Key #8).

Obviously you can't be aware of everything all the time. It's impossible! But just like strengthening the muscles of your body, the more attention you put on strengthening your awareness in particular areas, the more easily you'll have access to the data that is there for you to receive. You are a whole being, and the feedback you are receiving, however it comes (as a physical symptom, a strong emotion, a shift in your state of being), is all interwoven as guidance for you. The wide-open territory of YOU and your body-home is there for you to learn about. The important thing is simply to begin. You gather the feedback that your innate inner wisdom—your life-energy—is sharing with you so that you can garden yourself into the most alive, vital version of you that you can be.

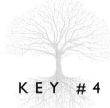

CULTIVATING RESILIENCE

✦

"You cannot control what happens to you, but you can control your attitude toward what happens to you, and in that, you will be mastering change rather than allowing it to master you."
—BRIAN TRACY

"WHAT DO I DO with all of this information?"

James, a fifty-four-year-old graphic designer living in Seattle, sat across from me, drumming his fingers on the table. Had I looked under the table I'm sure I would have seen him tapping his foot as well. While he already looked visibly less exhausted and stressed than he had in our initial sessions, he was clearly finding it difficult to stay in the increasing awareness that we'd been working on in Key #3.

"I warned you it might be uncomfortable here!" I reminded him with a smile. "But don't worry—you don't have to stay here forever. You've uncovered so much important data these past few weeks; now you're ready to learn how to use it."

James had initially come to see me because he felt depleted and exhausted. "I have such a hard time getting going in the morning, and I'm not sleeping well at night. I just don't have the energy to do the things I love to do," he told me in our first meeting. James was an avid outdoorsman and loved to hike and travel. He also enjoyed dancing, live music, and theater, but now he felt no energy for any of these passions.

"I feel depressed," he said, "because I am missing out on parts of my life. Feeling tired all the time makes my days no fun. And then I feel anxious and overwhelmed, too, because it always seems like there is more to do than

I have the energy or time for. I'd like to understand how to better care for myself so that I can work with the energy that I do have and learn how to increase it. I want to come to understand how my daily habits might not be serving me and to learn some things that I can do to make a difference."

Now, after several weeks of paying close attention to his daily habits and the ways in which they affected his vitality, I asked James what he'd learned.

"I'm able to see with clearer eyes and be honest about some of my patterns that aren't supporting me," he said. "My irregular sleep habits, for instance, are something I have not directly faced, despite my experience of exhaustion! I often go to bed at 2:30 a.m. and wake up at 8:00 a.m. to go to work, and assume that I ought to be fine. Or I might occasionally use marijuana or eat large amounts of cake in the evenings—I didn't realize that these might be numbing behaviors that are having the effect of disrupting my sleep and keeping me disconnected from feeling myself more authentically. I think that before we began our work, I didn't want to admit to myself that these choices might be having a huge impact on my energy levels.

"I feel like I'm starting to listen to what my body is trying to tell me in terms of my health and well-being. And I've just been staying there, as you suggested. But now I feel ready to make some changes."

LEARNING THE SKILLS OF RESILIENCE

The fourth key, Cultivating Resilience, is intimately connected to and builds on the third. Awareness, on this path, is not something we develop for its own sake—it is a tool with which we can create informed change in our behaviors, habits, and experiences. As the psychologist Mihaly Csikszentmihalyi writes in his seminal work *Flow*, "The function of consciousness is to represent information about what is happening inside and outside the organism in such a way that it can be evaluated and acted upon by the body." And he points out that "the human nervous system has become so complex that it is now able to affect its own states."[40]

Key #4 helps you begin to engage with all of the feedback you receive and use it to affect your state of being. I have chosen the term "resilience" because it reflects an important reality: you are not a static entity, but an evolving, changing being in a rapidly changing environment. Any approach to your health and well-being that denies this critical fact will always fall short. As ecologists Brian Walker and David Salt write in *Resilience Thinking*, "At the heart of resilience thinking is a very simple notion—things change—and to ignore or resist this change is to increase our vulnerability and forego emerging opportunities. In so doing, we limit our options."[41]

They go on to define resilience as "the capacity of a system to absorb disturbance; to undergo change and still retain essentially the same function, structure, and feedbacks."

Resilience, in the way I use the term, is an inner orientation, the way you view yourself in relationship to your life, and, most importantly, it is about learning and honing the skills and capacities you need to consciously guide yourself toward your own flourishing in the midst of ongoing change.

Life is unpredictable and complex. You may be going along and feeling like you are on top of the world, and then suddenly, you are in a car accident, or a loved one dies, or you lose your job. All of a sudden, just like that, everything changes. There is no such thing as a stress-free or predictable life.

When things like that happen, it can feel like the ground beneath you drops out, and there is no sense of control or security. And on one level that is true. You really do not ultimately have control over what happens. Death, loss, and change are all part of life's unfolding. What you do have control over, however, is how you respond within the unpredictability and the constant change. Through developing resilience, you can self-regulate and preserve your health and well-being even when life throws you a curveball.

UNDERSTANDING THE STRESS-RESPONSE CASCADE

As we've already discussed in this book, stress is a big deal. The sources of it are varied (and unique to each of us), yet every single person I have ever worked with had stress as a central contributor to the *dis*-ease they experienced in their lives. It feels important, therefore, to start off our exploration of cultivating resilience by bringing stress (and the skills and capacities we can learn to shift our experience of stress) front and center. Later in the chapter we will talk about a whole range of other skills, knowledge, and approaches to help us build our resilience.

I'd like you to play along with me here and think of all of the different things that stress you out in your life now—your physical health, relationships, family, work, finances, the state of the world, sex, community, your love life, responsibilities, etc. You might pause for a few minutes and even do a stream-of-consciousness writing exercise in your journal to explore what comes up. Allow yourself to really feel it all in this moment and notice what happens in your body.

Perhaps you started sweating, or noticed that your heart rate increased. Maybe your hands and feet got a bit colder, or you got a sense of discomfort in your gut. Maybe you started breathing a bit faster. Sometimes, even just the thought of something stressful can send us spiraling down what is known as the stress-response cascade. I don't want you to stay in a stress response now, so before you read on you might want to calm yourself with a minute of slow breathing (try breathing in to the count of five and breathing out to the count of five) and see what happens. Feel calmer? Congratulations, you just did a mini-version of what I'll be teaching you in this chapter.

When a stress trigger happens, it can often feel like we have no control over our responses. Our bodies are designed to respond to stress with what's known as a "fight-or-flight" response. When a stressful event (including a thought or series of thoughts) happens, it triggers both the cerebral cortex of the brain and the amygdala, which is part of the limbic system. The cerebral cortex is what we consider the higher, developed, rational, thinking part of our brain. This is the part that is able to consciously assess whether there is a need to be stressed or not. If there is a need to be stressed, the cerebral cortex causes the release of chemicals in our brain to heighten our mental awareness. If not, we simply come to the conclusion that everything is all right and the feedback is sent to shut down the other reactions that are already happening. Although your rational cortex may give the feedback to your body that there is no need to be stressed, you may find yourself already in a full-blown stress response and experience quite a delay in reversing the effects of that. Why? Because the amygdala, which is part of the more primitive, emotional response center of the brain, was triggered by that stressful event, too. And the amygdala sends the signal on to the hypothalamus, a control center in the brain linked to both the nervous system and the endocrine (hormonal) system. The hypothalamus sends the stress-alert signal to the sympathetic nervous system. This triggers a very rapid "fight or flight" response in the body—adrenaline is pumped into our system. All the symptoms that I mentioned above—an increase in sweating, an increase in heart rate, a dilation of the bronchi allowing more oxygen into the lungs, cold hands and feet, pupils dilating, and a decrease in digestive function—are all direct results of the activated sympathetic nervous system.

Essentially, it tells your body to prioritize the organs and systems that will help you get the hell out of an emergency situation. You don't need to be digesting your food or having all of your blood flowing to your extremities when you are about to be attacked—you need to be able to run fast and make sure your essential organs have all the blood they need. Yet you can also see how, if you are in a chronic-stress situation in which your sympathetic nervous system is increasingly activated, it could have significant negative impacts; for instance, your digestive system can become comprised.

Remember, the hypothalamus is also connected to the endocrine system. It sends on the stress alert to the pituitary gland, which sends it on to the adrenal cortex, which releases the hormone cortisol, and to the thyroid, which releases the hormone thyroxine. While the sympathetic nervous system kicks in almost immediately with all of the stress-response symptoms, the endocrine system is slower to respond and cause its effects, but it also lasts longer. So in chronic stress, cortisol levels can be elevated, circulating at times of the day that they wouldn't normally be, disrupting our sleep and stimulating us in ways that can be very confusing. Likewise, if the thyroid gland is overstimulated in this way, it can grow tired and depleted over time, causing hypothyroidism, a common condition in this day and age.

I know that that was a lot of biochemistry and physiology that I just shared. I did so to give you a window into some of the territory that you may want to study more. Beginning to learn about how our responses to stressful triggers play out in our bodies can help us to link our growing awareness of what is happening with an understanding of *why* it is happening. Add to this knowledge new skills that can help us reverse the stress cascade, and we become empowered in our self-care—an extraordinary attainment in our stressed-out world.

Whether your stress comes from a devastating loss or simply from challenges in your everyday life, you have the capacity to learn how to shift your response on every level—physically, mentally, emotionally, and spiritually. When stressors come (and they will come!), you are able to consciously adapt and steer yourself back to a more alive, vital place. You discover a ground inside of yourself that is always there to solidly stand on, even when it feels like life has dropped out from under you.

In other words, Cultivating Resilience is about recognizing that you have the capacity to learn the skills to self-regulate, to realign and redirect your state of being on all levels at any moment. It is about heeding the feedback you are receiving, the data that your expanding self-awareness makes available to you, and directing yourself accordingly.

USING BIOFEEDBACK

For James, applying the Cultivating Resilience key meant studying and adjusting his patterns around sleep, nutrition, and other lifestyle habits. First, I introduced him to the concept of "biofeedback." Neuroscientist David S. Olton and psychologist Aaron R. Noonberg, in their book *Biofeedback: Clinical Applications in Behavioral Medicine*, define biofeedback "as any technique which increases the ability of a person to control voluntary physiological activities by providing information about those activities."[42] In a broad sense, biofeedback is a term for our capacity to receive feedback about how our body is responding and then to consciously shift that response using learned skills. It's an ongoing process, a feedback loop, of receiving the data and then adjusting.

Typically this happens through objective data that we gather through the use of sensors and computer programs that track things like heart rate and variability, breath rate and depth, skin temperature and moisture, muscle tension, blood pressure, and more. As discussed in the previous chapter, it can be incredibly helpful to see your body's data in an objective way, heightening your self-awareness of how your body responds to different stimuli and what your habitual baselines may actually be.

When beginning to use biofeedback with clients, I watch their shock when they see firsthand how intimately linked the body's responses are to a single thought, a manner of breathing, or an emotional state. It becomes undeniable that no part of us is separate from any other part—what's going on in the shadows is mirrored in our bodies; what's happening with our breath ripples out into our emotional states, and vice versa. Using biofeedback to cultivate resilience allows us to consciously embrace our complexity as human beings and to truly begin to treat ourselves as a whole person. Every choice we make impacts all aspects of ourselves.

While electronic sensors and computer programs can be incredibly helpful as we begin to get the hang of how to strengthen our self-awareness muscles and consciously steer ourselves, they are not necessary. Biofeedback can happen without the computerized data. As we discussed in the previous key, you can learn a ton from noticing how your body feels, how your stools look, what your energy level is, and how your mood fluctuates. These simple awarenesses can give you the necessary feedback to guide you on your journey toward deep vitality.

For James, the tools and the computer program were really helpful. I taught him how to use simple breathing exercises to regulate stress, and the monitor tracked his heart-rate variability, a highly sensitive marker that is used to track the state of the nervous system (so highly sensitive, in fact, that it is used in lie-detector tests!). "I'm a visual person so it allowed me to experience more deeply how I was breathing and how that was influencing the state of my nervous system," he told me, after working with the tools for a few weeks. "I was able to engage more fully with my senses and to tune in more deeply to the natural cycles that I could influence. I was able to learn how to breathe more optimally in a way to bring myself into a state of relaxation quite quickly and to feel what it is to really let go with my exhale."

James said that after a few months, he felt like he had reconnected to his natural rhythm, content with the pacing of his body. "I felt integrated," he said. "It wasn't an anxious super-charged energy, but a healthy flowing energy. I learned that my body has a natural rhythm that I can get out of sync with all the time in my daily life. Yet with the breathing exercises I came to see that I can always come back to it whenever I need to."

THE REGULATING POWER OF BREATH

Most of us have not been taught optimal breathing. We breathe how we breathe and that's it. Yet your breath is an incredible, empowering doorway through which you can influence so much of your body's physiology. When you learn to optimally breathe (which for most of us these days means slowing down our breath and breathing more diaphragmatically), you can shift your nervous system out of a chronic, sympathetic (fight-or-flight) state, to a predominantly parasympathetic (rest-and-relax) state. This is a critical skill for self-regulation that can impact how you feel on every level, and how your entire body functions—from digestion, to sleep, to muscle tension, to your moods, to a number of chronic illnesses.

In the biofeedback work and the breath retraining I did with James, our focus was on using the breath to help him shift out of anxiety and exhaustion into a relaxed and energized state. When we first began working together, I noticed that he was breathing predominantly from his chest, and that his breath rate was quite fast. This is a common pattern when people are in more of a sympathetic nervous system state. I often initially have folks put one hand on their chests and one hand on their abdomens as a way to strengthen their awareness around where they are breathing from.

I focused on helping James to consciously shift his breathing into his diaphragm and abdomen. You can get a feel for this by interlacing your fingers and raising your arms above your head, palm side up. If you breathe like this you will notice that it is almost impossible to breathe from your chest in this position. Your breath will naturally shift to your abdomen. You can do this for about a minute and then slowly drop your arms to your sides and see if you can maintain your breathing from that place.

You can also try placing your hands on your lower ribs, fingers forward, your thumbs looped onto your back. As you breathe in, consciously push out against your hands, and as you breathe out, gently push your hands toward each other. Again repeat this for about a minute and then drop your hands and notice what has changed for you. With a simple Google search, you will find numerous exercises you can learn that help strengthen your diaphragm and help loosen and stimulate your natural breathing patterns, including yoga movements and simple stretching exercises.

In addition to learning to breathe abdomino-diaphragmatically, there is also the issue of breath rate. Most people breathe much more rapidly than is optimal for their body systems. This reinforces a chronic stress state in the body. Slowing down your breath rate is a powerful tool that you can use anytime and anywhere. While there are more nuanced ways to assess your optimal breath rate that can be discovered using biofeedback, the majority of people optimally fall between 5 and 7 breaths per minute (versus the 12 to 20 breaths per minute that medical professionals are standardly taught).[43, 44] Simply put, if you practice breathing in to a count of five and breathing out to a count of five you will land somewhere in the right ballpark for an optimal breath rate, around 6 breaths per minute. I use this practice at night in bed to help me to relax into falling asleep. It is simple enough that you can do it in the car while driving, or at work at your desk. And there are of course an abundance of apps available for your smartphone or computer that can guide you in slowing down your breath. In other words, you can practice optimal breathing anywhere.

With James, I used all of these practices and tools in combination with HeartMath, a wonderful and effective biofeedback program available on handheld devices as well as on your computer, and easy to understand for folks without any special training or medical background.

When I asked James to reflect on his learning and the impact that the whole set of tools we used had, he said, "Before doing the breathing exercises, I would feel tired and anxious at the same time. My body felt heavy, and I was drudging along. And then there was the anxious part that felt like I needed to plow through the day regardless. In my body, I came to recognize that it was like my head and chest were trying to pull me along, while the rest of my body was this huge tired weight. It felt as if the anxious me was a mouse trying to tow a car. The anxious part was geared up to pull really hard, yet it wasn't in alignment with what was behind it.

"I was really amazed," he continued, "how it didn't take long to learn how to sync my breath with my own natural rhythm, to optimize my breathing to relax and come more fully home to myself. It just felt like riding a bike and changing speeds. Before, it was as if the derailleur wasn't quite in place and was grinding a bit. But once I did the exercises and got in sync more, it was like the gears were running really well. They were aligned in a way that felt fluid and natural. These breathing exercises were very empowering, especially when coupled with the realizations you helped me come to about my daily patterns."

SKILL BUILDING AND SELF-EDUCATION

The optimal breathing practice described above is just one type of skill that helps to cultivate resilience. The collection of things we can do all on our own is never ending. We can learn about nutrition and identify the foods that resonate best with our bodies; discover the things that best promote rejuvenating sleep; learn how to release tension in our bodies (before it even becomes tension!); feel, integrate, and consciously release emotional reactions; listen to and heed our intuition and inner guidance; and so much more!

All of these things impact our state of vitality and aliveness all the time.

Once you begin to consciously receive the feedback (as we learned in Key #3), you then have the opportunity to apply the things you are learning in ways that feel congruent and aligned for you. On the surface, many of the skills might seem similar to what you are already doing—you might take a cooking class, or have a strength trainer help you out at the gym. But the difference is this: When you are learning these skills in the context of your own expanding self-awareness, you no longer have to shoot in the dark or blindly follow someone else's protocol. Instead you are seeking out what you most need to learn so you can more lovingly and skillfully guide yourself toward your own thriving.

You will also find that your newfound knowledge and improved ability to self-regulate brings with it a heightened sense of self-awareness—a consciousness that will inevitably help you make more informed choices. You can expand your capacities and feel confident in these skills so that you have a sense of strength within, an increased aptitude for transforming yourself and actively shifting your trajectory in response to the constant feedback your body is providing you.

Cultivating resilience involves a lot of active learning—the acquisition of concrete skills and information, as well as a shift in your orientation, beliefs, and capacities. The learning begins with acknowledging that you very well might be a beginner in much of this territory. Not only does embracing the orientation of being a beginner allow you to open more fully with curiosity to the third key, Strengthening Your Self-Awareness Muscles, but it also allows you to seek out the skills training that will support you in cultivating resilience—without apology, self-judgment, or urgency.

In this chapter, we are just scratching the surface of what's possible for you. But the point of this key is for you to discover for yourself what works and what doesn't. It's not my place to tell you, or anyone else's place for that matter. That being said, it is quite likely that you will need help from others as you develop these capacities. You can seek out practitioners, groups, programs, or books that can help you begin to develop the skills to self-regulate. And as you reach out, it will come from an attitude of proactive self-responsibility, of being an empowered author of your own vitality. You can start to see your doctors as teachers who support you on your journey, not as mechanics who are there to fix you or solve your problems. Did you know that the word root of doctor is "docere," which means to teach? This, to me, is the real heart of medicine—teaching people how to cultivate the awareness and skills to feel empowered in guiding themselves toward their own thriving.

In *When the Body Says No*, Gabor Maté agrees that there is no true responsibility without awareness:

> One of the weaknesses of the Western medical approach is that we have made the physician the only authority, with the patient often a mere recipient of the treatment or cure. People are deprived of the opportunity to become truly responsible. None of us are to be blamed if we succumb to illness and death. Any one of us might succumb at any time, but the more we can learn about ourselves, the less prone we are to become passive victims.[45]

When you begin to cultivate resilience, your health journey is no longer about a long externally created list of all the things you "should" be doing in order to be healthy. Instead, your journey becomes about learning skills and expanding your awareness so that you can truly embrace being in charge of YOU!

Here's another benefit: the unconscious ways in which you may feel like a victim when it comes to your health drop away. This seems to me to be part of our cultural paradigm around health. I heard myself say recently, "I got sick last week, and I can't seem to get better." Sure, on one level these statements were accurate. And yet can you hear the subtle victim orientation there? It was like something had taken me over and I had no control or power anymore. No wonder, at moments like that, that we want to go to a doctor who can simply fix us and make us better.

Language is such a powerful mirror for what is going on in our unconscious, for what's happening in the shadows that is running the show without us being aware. So if we're telling ourselves things like, "I can't lose this weight," or "I can't fall asleep," or "I guess I should just get used to not feeling well and accept that that's how it is going to be from now on," we may be perpetuating a reality that we do in fact have the power to shift.

If you begin to view your experiences, even the painful ones, not as ailments but as feedback, you'll quickly stop feeling like a victim. Symptoms are like nudges, or guideposts, to help to move you toward greater alignment and aliveness, and into a higher state of vitality and wellness.

CHECKING IN: *We've reviewed so much during this chapter so far, and I just want to encourage you to pause here for a minute. How are you feeling in your body right now? What might be something you could do for yourself in this moment that would bring more ease? What would help you integrate your learning here in a gentle, loving way?*

IDEAS FOR CULTIVATING RESILIENCE

The following are some areas in which you might begin to focus on cultivating resilience. With each area, I will simply provide some suggestions of skills you might want to work with or things you might study—an initial taste of what may be possible for you. Obviously this is just the beginning of a lifetime exploration, and what is right for one person will be different from what is right for another. Allow your self-awareness to guide you as you read through these examples and see which feel relevant and resonant for you.

YOUR ANATOMY & PHYSIOLOGY: Unless you have trained as a health professional of some kind, chances are you have never studied the anatomy and physiology of the human body. Learning about the body—its skeletal makeup, its systems, and how it functions—is incredibly empowering. No longer is your body foreign—you can begin to visualize where your organs are and how you are structured. Add to that an understanding of how each of your body systems works, and you have a much less mysterious context to gather feedback from, feedback you can use to consciously support yourself. When your body sends a message of pain, for example, you'll know, sometimes exactly, where that pain is coming from, and what organs and influences are involved. And when you hear the latest study about what you should do, eat, follow, or supplement your diet with in order to be healthy, you will have a more comprehensive understanding of how that theory relates to how your body works. Local community colleges have classes you can sign up for, and of course there are a plethora of anatomy and physiology books available—I recommend ones with lots of pictures!

STRUCTURAL INTEGRITY & FLEXIBILITY: Part of understanding the anatomy and physiology of your body includes understanding how your body's structure—your spine, your bones, your joints, the fascia covering them, and your muscles—supports the optimal functioning of your body. The nerves come out of your spinal cord and innervate your organs and every part of your body. Supporting the optimal alignment of your spine and the flexibility and fluidity of movement in your joints allows for the nerves to do their best job communicating with the various parts of your body. You can learn a lot on this topic from yoga instructors, massage therapists, chiropractors, osteopaths, craniosacral practitioners, and other bodyworkers.

DIGESTION, NUTRITION, & EATING: If you did the diet diary exercise in the last chapter you likely now have some more awareness around what you are eating, how you are digesting it, and how the foods you are taking in make you feel. With this kind of awareness, you are primed to take proactive steps toward more learning and to experiment and observe in order to get clearer feedback. This is a great time to use your discernment to explore the different nutritional theories out there. See which ones philosophically resonate for you and make sense and then try them out for periods of time to see how they make you feel. The key is not to get attached to the theory, approach, or diet in and of itself, but to find the mix of foods that works best for you.

I'd suggest starting with a basic nutrition class (one with a whole-foods emphasis if possible!) so that you can really understand the different types of nutrients and food groups. That way, when you are assessing the different diet theories, you will have a strong base of knowledge to use alongside your own body-home's feedback. If you find yourself easily overwhelmed with all the information out there, I'm a big fan of keeping it super simple. As author Michael Pollan writes in his book *In Defense of Food: An Eater's Manifesto*, "Don't eat anything your great grandmother wouldn't recognize as food."[46]

These are some basic guidelines that I use in my eating:

◆ Stick with whole foods

◆ Try to have half my plate at meals be vegetables

◆ See if I can eat all the colors of the rainbow each day

◆ Avoid (as much as possible) processed foods, additives, and any ingredients that do not directly come from a whole food

◆ Eat organic, non-GMO, and local as much as I can—these foods have a higher nutrient content, are better for the sustainability of agricultural land and culture, and don't expose me to harmful chemicals found in common pesticides and herbicides.

Another area to explore that can have a huge impact on vitality is the realm of food sensitivities, intolerances, and allergies. This topic is too large to do justice to in the context of this book, but I wanted to introduce it into your awareness. You can easily begin this exploration on your own, yet if you want to dive deeper into it, I'd strongly encourage you to seek out professional support with a licensed naturopathic physician or a holistically trained nutritionist. I suggest this as it can spare you a lot of grief, confusion, and possibly eating disorders—all of which can develop when you become afraid of how the foods you are eating might be affecting you. The goal, whichever path you take to get there, is to feel empowered to guide yourself toward your own vitality, not to guide yourself into new neuroses!

You might begin to pay attention to whether there are particular foods that your body-home doesn't seem to do well with (your diet diary may have some insights for you). Perhaps your energy dips after you eat them, or you have intense cravings, or you get bloated or have diarrhea. Or you might have more extreme symptoms like migraines, blood-sugar instability, depression, or rashes. It can be hard sometimes to tell which food might be at the root of the symptoms. You can play around with identifying the key culprit(s) and then doing a simple complete elimination of that food from your diet for a few weeks, see how you feel without it, then see what happens when you eat it again.

If you suspect that certain foods might be a significant contributor to your symptoms, again I'd suggest getting professional support and perhaps trying a more complete elimination diet (also sometimes called an anti-inflammatory diet protocol). This will give you a support structure (and help in knowing what symptoms to look for) as you eliminate multiple foods at once and then reintroduce them in a controlled, systematic way one at a time to get feedback about which of those foods may not be such a resonant fit for you.

Common foods that cause difficulty for people in modern-day Western culture are wheat (and sometimes all gluten grains), dairy, corn, eggs, soy, sugar, alcohol, caffeine, and citrus. Again, I want to emphasize that this is not about looking for what's wrong and creating a sense of pathology for yourself; it is about having greater discernment and self-knowledge to support your flourishing. I see so many folks hopping on the "gluten-free" bandwagon these days because it is "the thing" to do to be healthy; they end up limiting their diet, and eating lots of processed gluten-free foods as substitutes when they might not even have a gluten sensitivity at all.

There are so many factors that influence our food choices and preferences, and so many reasons that certain foods will resonate best with our particular bodies. These factors include our genetics, cultural heritage, location and climate, occupation and lifestyle, activity level, age, constitutional type, and particular food allergies and sensitivities. Cultivating resilience in this realm is taking charge of discovering and aligning with what is true for you.

YOUR THOUGHTS & EMOTIONS: One of the powerful things that you can see immediately when exploring with biofeedback tools is that your thoughts and emotions have big physiological impacts on your body at every moment. When you consciously cultivate the capacity to shift your mental and emotional states through meditation, visualization, or relaxation techniques, you can immediately shift the physiology of your body and, through ongoing cultivation, you can shift the baseline norms of your body's system to a predominantly relaxed state.

This is where HeartMath and other biofeedback programs can be very eye-opening and helpful in giving you greater clarity. They can help you determine how the practices you are using are supporting (or not supporting) your body's state of being. In their insightful book *The HeartMath Solution*, Doc Childre, founder of the HeartMath Institute, and Howard Martin write that "our mental and emotional diets determine our overall energy levels, health, and well-being to a far greater extent than most people realize."[47] You can experiment with activating heart-opening emotions like appreciation, gratitude, and love to shift your body's physiological state and to create a more practiced agility in moving from stressful thoughts and emotions back to a foundation of ease and relaxation.

The objective physiological monitoring of a biofeedback device can provide surprising insight. I have seen even longtime meditators be taken aback when they see what is actually happening in their body's systems. One's own subjective assessment of one's state of being often does not match what is objectively happening. Yet with a little bit of outside input, you can recalibrate your subjective experience. Even monitoring your pulse or blood pressure before and after you use a relaxation technique can be a great place to start.

When learning to shift your state in relationship to your thoughts and emotions, it is important to realize that this isn't about suppression or avoidance. Nothing you are feeling or thinking is bad or wrong. When you are willing to fully embrace your experience and without judgment feel and acknowledge what's true for you, you can let go much more easily.

To experiment with shifting your emotional and mental states, you can take advantage of the plethora of different meditation, mindfulness, and yoga classes out there. I'm a big fan of dancing, too, to connect with what you are feeling and to move emotions through your body. Using your voice to move sound, express your emotions, and sing is another way to shift your internal state.

You can also try experimenting with how your body posture changes your mood. What happens when you walk around bent slightly over, versus standing tall with your eyes looking ahead and your chest out? What happens when you put your face in the expression of a smile, even if you don't feel happy? You might want to try some laughter therapy; when you *make* yourself laugh, your body's physiology can respond in the same ways as it would with natural spontaneous laughter.

YOUR SLEEP: I can't emphasize enough the influence that sleep has on your state of vitality. I hear so often from friends, colleagues, and clients that they sacrifice sleep in order to prioritize other life responsibilities. To say that you can get by on only five hours of sleep has become, culturally, a thing to brag about. While there is a range of what different people need in regard to sleep, it can't be denied that sleep, for all of us, is a vital time of regeneration and restoration in our bodies—detoxification processes, muscle building, breakdown of fats, normalization of blood sugar, release of growth hormone, and so much more happen during this time. And according to a study from the Walter Reed Army Institute of Research, sleep deprivation reduces our ability to manage stress and impulse control; decreases our capacity for empathy; undermines the quality of our interpersonal relationships; diminishes our self-regard, assertiveness, and sense of independence; and hinders positive thinking and action, among other things.[48]

If sleep is something you struggle with, or you simply never feel rested and energetic (without drinking lots of coffee or other caffeinated beverages), there are skills you can utilize to shift your patterns. Here are a few examples to give you a taste, yet this may be an area in which to seek out some personalized professional guidance and support to get at the root of what may be preventing you from getting restorative sleep.

The number one shift you can make when it comes to changing your sleeping patterns is a mental shift: giving yourself full permission to let your body sleep as much as it needs in order to let you feel rested (yes, to actually wake feeling rested!). Some people need nine hours a night on a regular basis. Listen to your body's feedback, not your brain's or culture's idea of what is supposed to be enough.

Second, try making your bed and bedroom a place that feels really comfortable, cozy, and that lulls you into sleep. Reserve that room for sleep and sex only, if possible. Reduce clutter. Keep it dark. Remove electronic devices from around the bed. Try to have time before you go to sleep that is away from any electronic screens. Try to maintain consistent sleep and wake times. Listen to your body and notice when it first starts to get tired; prepare yourself for sleep then, and don't wait until you feel you are nodding off or the second wind comes. An evening and bedtime routine can be super helpful, one that lets your body know that you are relaxing into sleep time. A bath, meditation, cuddle time with your partner, breathing exercises, reading a book—all of these can be gentle ways to ease into a restful and restorative night's sleep.

RELAXATION & PLAY: As strange as it sounds, authentic play and relaxation may be skills you need to learn. Much of what we call "downtime" these days can take the form of more of a surface-level comfort or a social obligation, rather than an activity or level of rest that deeply restores. In fact, I consider this so important that we'll be returning to it as a central theme in Key #6. For now, I'd strongly encourage you to experiment with weaving play and deep soul-nourishing relaxation into each day. Don't think of it as a "should," where the play gets co-opted into being yet another thing to do (or feel guilty about not doing). Try to embrace the spirit of "I get to do ___!!" like a young child ecstatic at the joy of being alive and getting to play. A nap in the sun. A slow meandering walk with a dear friend. Swinging on a swing at the local playground. Renting a kayak for the afternoon. You know what you love to do and what brings you that exuberant, joyful, openhearted feeling inside. Go and do it, with no need for justification or excuses. This is your birthright!

EXERCISE: Just as with diet, the realm of exercise can really trip people up these days with all of the theories of what you should and shouldn't be doing. Here's how I see it: As human animals, we are designed to be active and to move. Modern society has many of us being remarkably sedentary and, as a result, many health struggles ensue. I'd encourage you to start with finding activities that you enjoy, so that you come to look forward to moving your body. You can let go of the associations you have with "exercise." Forget about what you "should" be doing and do what you love.

If running on a treadmill bores you to tears, but competitive sports light up your energy and vitality, get out of the gym and join a local team. Make it social. Try new things. Incorporate time outside in nature. Have fun! Dance! Once you find a regular rhythm in which you love moving your body, then you can expand and explore new realms that might add in some specific strengthening or aerobic capacity that you hadn't developed otherwise. Take it one step at a time, and stay aligned with your truth.

SEXUALITY: In the previous chapter, I touched on how crazy it is that something so fundamental to our vitality (and life!) as sex is largely neglected in health conversations. Nurturing and moving sexual energy on a regular basis, regardless of whether you are romantically inclined, in a relationship or not, is absolutely foundational to your health and well-being. Opening to this natural pleasure and self-nourishment will free up your life-energy in all areas of your life.

A phrase that one of my mentor teachers once said has stuck in my head: "An orgasm a day keeps the doctor away!" It seems like a very pleasurable experiment to try, doesn't it? I don't say this to reduce sex to chasing orgasms; what I am pointing to is that our vitality is deeply nourished through opening to feel, experience, and stay in contact with the primal pleasure of our sexual creative life-force. Saying yes to this foundational life-energy on a regular basis is, to me, akin to saying yes to life itself.

So whether you are single or in a relationship, sexually experienced or

newly discovering, I encourage you to explore your sexuality as a relationship with yourself that needs constant nourishment, new growth, and spice.
Buy yourself a sexy novel or a how-to sex guide. Go online or take yourself
to a local sex shop (the kind that feels safe, educational, and positive) and
buy yourself some new supplies and toys. Learn new ways to connect with
yourself or a partner in pleasure and sexual ecstasy. And don't be shy to
reach out for support. This is an area ripe with shame and shadows for so
many of us.

ATTENTION: If you've noticed that your attention tends to be scattered
and you're always multitasking, you might want to experiment with ways
to focus yourself and develop the capacity to do only one thing at a time
(which some people call "unitasking"). A recent article in *Forbes* cites several
prominent research studies that suggest that multitasking may actually be
quite harmful to us. Researchers at Stanford have shown that it is not as productive as focusing on one thing at a time. They also found that people who
regularly multitask with technologies can't switch from one undertaking to
another, recall details, or pay attention as well as those who typically focus
on doing one thing at a time. Another research study at the University of
London has actually shown that multitasking lowers the IQ, much akin to
getting no sleep. At the University of Sussex, researchers are looking at MRI
scans of people who tend to multitask by using more than one technological device at the same time, revealing that this habit can result in structural
changes in our brains, potentially causing a type of brain damage.[49]

As our lives become more and more tied to technology, many people are
finding it helpful to create "technology-free" periods during their days or
weeks, or even doing "technology detoxes." I'm a huge fan of spending time
in nature as a way to ground the frenetic attention and awaken a remembrance of the simplicity at the heart of life. It feels like it reconnects me to a
bigger view and puts the attention-grabbing busyness in that larger context,
refocusing my attention like nothing else.

You may also want to turn to the most ancient human technology for
clearing and focusing your attention: meditation. There are so many different styles, traditions, and approaches to meditation that I will leave it to
you to explore what resonates and brings benefit to your life. Some types
feel akin to strengthening the muscle of focus and attention, honing your
capacity to stay attuned to one thing in all of its intricate sensual detail.

Other types help you to widen the embrace of your attention and relax into being present to the whole array of what is arising at any given moment through all of your perceptual and sensory channels—simply noticing without changing anything.

ELIMINATION PATHWAYS: Our kidneys, large intestine, bowels, liver, skin, lymphatic system, and lungs are all involved with helping our bodies to process and let go of what we no longer need. Learning how to optimally support that process is vital to our ongoing health. What's needed is much simpler than all of the fancy and expensive "detox" programs out there. The learning here is about what we're doing in our daily life, not about needing to do a "cleanse" once a year.

One of the simplest and most important factors is adequate hydration. A recent Harvard study showed that over half of children and adolescents in the United States are not adequately hydrated![50] Other examples of simple daily nourishment for the elimination pathways include helping the body to sweat regularly, physical movement, eating whole foods that bring natural fiber into the diet, and receiving massage and other bodywork. The elimination pathways are a rich area to focus your learning around anatomy, physiology, and biochemistry; helping the body to optimally release what we no longer need is a vital yet often underappreciated part of self-nourishment.

I hope you are starting to recognize and connect with the wide-open territory of YOU and your body-home and its potential as a place for you to consciously develop your expertise and informed self-guidance. Don't be daunted by the task—the more you pursue it, the more you will find your natural interest taking over and energizing you.

To offer you a bit of encouragement as you embark on cultivating your resilience, here are the words of Saint Francis de Sales: "Have patience with all things, but chiefly have patience with yourself. Do not lose courage by considering your own imperfections, but instantly set about remedying them; every day begin the task anew."[51]

As you deepen your own self-knowing, you will discover an inherent ease and empowerment in caring for yourself. You will truly come to see yourself as your own primary healer. You will become masterful at guiding yourself, day in and day out, toward a state of optimal vitality.

ALIGNING WITH YOUR "YES!"

"Run my dear,
From anything
That may not strengthen
Your precious budding wings"
—HAFIZ

WHAT BRINGS YOU ALIVE?

When do you feel a sense of deep alignment, like you are doing exactly what you are made for?

What cracks you open into a raw contact with life, where you feel awake, clear, and in touch with the full spectrum of your humanity?

These questions can sometimes be harder to answer than you might expect.

Key #5: Aligning with Your "Yes!" is about consciously steering yourself toward your own thriving. It is about saying "yes!" to life. It is about cultivating a new guidance system for how you move through your days, self-calibrated to your own vitality and joy.

This key reveals one of the strange conundrums that I encountered on my own healing journey, a pattern I've also come to recognize in my clients and loved ones. The conundrum is this: you would think that we would all naturally move toward our own thriving. *It feels good!* Why wouldn't we align with what brings us deeply, soulfully alive? Why wouldn't we joyfully embrace our "yes!"? And yet, we don't, at least, not consistently.

In observing nature, we can see that plants and other animals do it. Close your eyes and return to the gardening metaphor we explored in Key #1.

Those seeds you planted, when given the appropriate balance of nutrients, water, and sunlight, will flourish and thrive. They will extend their roots deeper into the earth to maximize their capacity to take in water. They will angle themselves toward the sun to receive more of the light they need. You don't see those plants in the garden turning away from the sun. You don't see animals that are thirsty turning away from water that's in front of them.

And yet, I see us humans doing this to ourselves, again and again. It may not be water or sunlight that we turn away from, but there are other things that we neglect to do that have a dramatic impact on our capacity to thrive.

Think for a moment about what you most love, what lights you up. Are those things woven into your daily life? What about your deepest yearnings and desires, the kinds of things that you may barely even acknowledge to yourself, let alone shout from the rooftops? These are your deep soul yearnings. They may seem like too much to ask for. Indeed, you may have concluded that it is not okay for you to have these things in your life.

Aligning with Your "yes!" is about feeling nourished on every level—feeling deeply alive. I'm not talking about the shallow, quick-fix kinds of comfort that make us feel good only temporarily. The kind of feeling good that I'm talking about, which comes from aligning with your "yes!," is about listening for the deeper truth underneath all of that. Deep alignment evokes the sense of thriving, coming alive, feeling juiced. It's that knowledge that "I'm in the right place, at the right time, doing what I'm here to do." You feel grounded and at home in yourself. Your life becomes rooted in a deep "yes!" You feel alive and grateful to be in direct contact with life. You are in touch with how exquisite it is to feel and be with the raw truth of all that is moving through you. This kind of alignment includes difficult emotions, pain, and tension. It can include illness and struggle. It is about being in direct, authentic contact with the wholeness of life. Nothing is denied. It is your truth and you are awake to it.

This may sound too good to be true, but I assure you, I believe wholeheartedly and sincerely that this is possible for each and every one of us. We can all cultivate access to that deeper sense of aliveness, even when we are navigating an illness or challenge. It can be too easy to read about things like this and feel that it is not for you. It is for you! Turning toward yourself with kindness, reverence, and a commitment to your thriving can happen whether or not you have an acute physical ailment, a chronic illness, or you are facing a life-threatening disease. It is about being authentically present with the whole of you. It is about honoring your unique life and the path you are on.

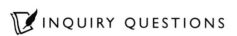 INQUIRY QUESTIONS

Grab your journal now and explore more about what it would mean to truly say "yes" to your "yes!" What would it mean for you to consciously create a life you love? Here are some questions to guide your exploration:

+ Let yourself open into a grand, playful, creative (unedited!) visioning process of what you would imagine your life to be—the who, whats, and wheres. With an openhearted curiosity, stand in your vitality and let it all come to you.

+ What makes you come most alive and how might you give yourself permission to integrate those things more fully, day to day?

+ If you get really honest with yourself and let go of any preconceived ideas you've had about yourself, what matters most to you in life?

+ What do you most yearn for? What are your deepest, most vulnerable desires?

+ How might you be closing yourself off from receiving what is right there being offered to you? Where might you be actively creating tension and *dis*-ease by not allowing yourself to open to let in a gift (someone or something) that would be very nurturing and life-giving for you?

+ What might you need to disentangle yourself from and let go of in order to open your heart to the possibilities and take steps toward them?

INVESTING YOUR LIFE-ENERGY

This key is about investing your life-energy where you get returns. When you, or your financial adviser, invest your money, I imagine you choose things that will give you a mixture of short-term and long-term returns. For the long-term investments, you might see some little dips here and there, but overall you will certainly want to see an increase in money, rather than a consistent decrease. It wouldn't be much of an investment if you lost money.

The same is true for your life-energy. When you invest your life-energy where there is a sense of alignment with why you are here, you get returns. In other words, you feel more vital and alive. And conversely, when out of alignment you will experience a lack of vitality, which manifests emotionally, psychologically, and even physically. When you unconsciously have your life-energy invested in things that are not a match for you and neglect the things you are here to do, it drains your life-energy away. You get symptoms and side effects of all kinds. You get no returns, and you lose energy in the process. The pioneering psychologist Abraham Maslow wrote, "A musician must make music, an artist must paint, a poet must write if he is to be ultimately at peace with himself. What a man can be, he must be."[52] And he noted that "if the essential core of the person is denied or suppressed, he gets sick sometimes in obvious ways, sometimes in subtle ways, sometimes immediately, sometimes later."[53] From what I have seen in myself and with my clients, denying yourself your true nature is a huge contributor to much of what plagues people in their health journeys.

As we discussed in Key #2: Facing and Embracing Your Shadows, the more you are in conscious direct contact with the whole of who you are, the easier it will be for you to consciously identify when you are out of alignment and to assess what might be contributing to that misalignment. And as you strengthen your self-awareness muscles, you will be able to feel and sense when something is bringing you more alive and when it is draining you. You will start to relate to the different elements of your life in terms of their cost or benefit to your life-energy. As Henry David Thoreau wrote, "The cost of a thing is the amount of what I call life which is required to be exchanged for it, immediately or in the long run."[54]

See if you can access, in your imagination, in a memory, or in your current lived experience, what it feels like to be aligned in this deepest, most profound way. How do you feel in your body? What shows up in your thoughts, in your emotional space? What's possible for your life when you stand in this experience of alignment? Can you name and make concrete the physical sensations, the emotions, the thoughts, the connection you feel to life, to something bigger than yourself?

When you are making choices that are in alignment with what deeply nourishes you, you get to feel the feedback of being more alive and present. And when you make choices that are not in alignment, then you get feedback of feeling disconnected from that sense of aliveness. I found this to be summed up so beautifully in a quotation I recently came across, which some attribute to an old Chinese proverb: "Tension is who you think you should be. Relaxation is who you are."

I saw an example of this all too clearly in a young woman I met a few years ago. When I first met Beth, she was finishing up a college degree in social work in Seattle, Washington. She seemed to be on fire with life and was one of the brightest, clearest, most awake young adults I had encountered. She clearly loved her studies and felt deeply aligned with her own vitality. But after her graduation, I noticed that the light that had seemed so very bright began to dim. When I asked her how she was feeling, she told me she was very stressed at work and experiencing all kinds of unpleasant physical symptoms. "My body feels like it is suffering," she said. "My periods have become painful, crampy, and intense. I've started to get migraines every couple of months; I throw up, and I break down and cry and go to bed. I feel like I have a lot of emotional energy pent up."

I sensed that for Beth, these symptoms were not just a physical ailment but a message from her body about where she'd gotten out of alignment in her life. I invited her to come on one of my mini vision-quest wilderness programs to see if she could get some clarity.

The weekend was powerful for Beth in many ways. What she realized was that she had come out of college and, within two weeks, started a job that turned out to be very stressful. "I remember feeling successful for being able to support myself," she said, "But now I realize that when I graduated college I was ready to get out of town and have some adventures. I didn't listen to that part of me." As a result, she had quickly become, as she put it, "cut off from very vital parts of myself." She couldn't remember the things that made her come alive, and she felt a strong urge to disconnect from home, work, and relationship, to run away. "I was bored, uninspired, disconnected," she said. "I felt as if my wings were clipped—I couldn't fly. I was trying to remember how, but my wings were sore and bruised. They'd been ignored for so long. *I* had been ignored for so long—by me."

The weekend helped Beth to rediscover her "yes!" and begin to look at what it would mean to bring her life into alignment. "I started to let go of all of the expectations I had for myself. I let it be okay to follow my heart again and go on an adventure. I remember thinking, 'Oh my gosh, I'm dreaming again!'" she said. "As I was walking back to the camp, I spontaneously found myself moving my arms up and down like I was flying. My wings were moving again."

In the several months that followed, Beth quit her job and, with the full support of her partner, set off on a series of adventures that included riding her bike down the West Coast and looking up long-lost relatives in other parts of the world. Now, after returning from her travels, she is about to embark on a new adventure: motherhood.

DON'T POSTPONE YOUR "YES!"

Beth was lucky that she came to this understanding so early in life. Don't let yourself wait another moment before you start engaging with this critical issue. It's not something you should put off until the kids leave home, or until you've made enough money, or until you retire. I've met many, many people who realize only when they reach their final years that they have spent a lifetime doing what they thought they "should" rather than what they truly loved and felt called to do. In fact, it's one of the most common deathbed regrets. Bronnie Ware, a hospice nurse who wrote the book *The Top Five Regrets of the Dying* after listening to hundreds of people in their final days, reported that the number one regret she heard was, "I wish I'd had the courage to live a life true to myself, not the life others expected of me."[55]

Reflecting on these men and women for whom it was now too late, Ware writes, "It is a pity that being who you truly are requires so much courage. But it does. . . . Being who you are, whatever it is, sometimes cannot even be articulated at first, even to yourself. All you know is there is a yearning within that is not being fulfilled by the life you are currently living."[56]

The good news is, unless you are truly taking your final breath, it's never too late. My client Laura was in her late fifties when, in the wake of her husband's death, she realized that she'd lost the thread of her own life and her own vitality. Somewhere on her journey as a mother, wife, and caregiver, she'd wandered away from herself. She said of that time, "So much of my life before was really tamped down in a lot of ways." She didn't waste any time getting started following her inner yearnings and, as a result, is more excited about life as she enters her sixties than she has been for decades.

Once you become committed to listening for and heeding your sense of yearning, however inarticulate it may be, everything changes. You are attuned beyond the surface level feedback, the quick fixes, the symptoms that go away with a pill. And you are listening for what it is that is really being asked of you in this lifetime. What choices may you need to reassess? What contexts are you rooted in that really may not be a fit for you any longer, or maybe never were? What are you saying "yes" to? What are you saying "no" to?

Alignment involves an ongoing intimate relationship with the feedback you are receiving. And the important thing here is that it is your internal feedback that will provide you with the support you need to create sustained change. When you become intimate with what is pointing you toward an alignment with your "yes!," you are able to pop out of all the externally created rules that you're surrounded by, all of the ideas and theories of what you are and aren't supposed to be doing to be healthy that you may constantly be trying to live up to. When you are aligned with your "yes!," there is an inner coherence on all levels that motivates you to continue to take care of yourself in those ways because it is not coming from a "should." It's coming from the deepest level of self-experience and knowledge. The wisdom of your life-energy is given free rein.

Once you really start to get an ongoing taste of what it feels like to align with your "yes!," there is no turning back. The other ways in which you may have tried to comfort or reward yourself in the past begin to reveal their true faces more quickly. You can't fool yourself any longer. Just as I discussed in Key #2: Facing and Embracing Your Shadows, this can be a painful transition. As you take the steps to align more fully with your "yes!," you can see how unconscious you may have been. How you may have justified the behavior patterns to yourself. How you may have denied yourself the experience of really coming alive. How you've lived in numbness. You may need to grieve in the midst of the openings and revelations. So again, as I've discussed before, as you transition in these ways, whatever it may look or feel like for you in your unique journey, please honor the tenderness of this and invite your inner Mama Bear to hold you, and seek out external support as well.

YOUR INNER GPS SYSTEM

Years ago, as I was beginning to consciously respond to this guidance from within, I described it to a friend as an inner GPS system. This analogy still feels apt. My inner GPS system is set to guide me toward my own thriving, or what brings me alive. The beautiful thing about a GPS is that at each step of the way it can tell you which way to go, and if you choose a different path or choice than what it tells you, it will simply recalibrate to your new location and guide you from there.

Aligning with your "yes!" isn't a linear path. You are far too complex and nuanced for that. There is no such thing as the perfect or "right" way. You are learning, evolving, and growing. What may feel aligned one day may feel like it no longer supports you a week later. So the GPS is a perfect guidance system because it has the capacity to recalibrate from where you are (and who you are) at any given time. Your "yes!" will change. What brings you alive will change. And yet your inner GPS knows that and can guide you accordingly. You simply set it for the orienting principle of "What will bring me alive?" and listen for what choice to make, what direction to go, and so on, as you encounter each decision in your life.

In other words, this key, Aligning with Your "Yes!," is about embracing a whole new guidance system for life that is rooted in the foundation you've been cultivating so far with the other four keys. This process involves both a masculine agency and a feminine receptivity at the same time. You are opening to receive the guidance, listening for who you truly are, and then taking the concrete steps to move yourself in the direction of what you are being guided toward.

Can you feel the incredible difference between this way of moving yourself on your health journey compared with a protocol someone gave you? When your guidance is all coming from outside of you, there is a pressure to stay on a narrow, linear path. When you stray off the path, you may beat yourself up about it, or give up, concluding that you can't achieve your goals. In the movement I'm describing, there is and can be no such thing as failure—only feedback to help you recalibrate and keep moving. You can't move toward a state of thriving, of feeling exquisitely alive, if you are doing so with rigidity and someone else's rulebook.

CHECKING IN: *Pause here for a minute and let all of what you have been reading sink in. How are you feeling in your body right now? What emotions are arising? What insights? What can you see about how your life-energy is invested now? Where are you getting returns, and where might you be unconsciously perpetuating a leaky bucket?*

PRUNING YOUR LIFE

In aligning with your "yes!," it's also important to learn to say "no." Have you ever pruned a fruit tree, or watched someone do it? It's a subtle and delicate process. You have to have discernment about which types of growth on the tree are unproductive. You also need to know how much to prune to optimize the growth. If you don't ever prune, the tree will not produce as much fruit and will become more and more unhealthy. The branches will be growing one on top of the next, blocking the sunlight from reaching the leaves and preventing the fruit from forming. And there will be an increasing number of what are called "suckers," branches that tend to grow straight up and never produce any fruit; they take the life-energy of the tree, but don't produce anything. Growth by itself is not all good. If not properly tended to and guided, the tree will become less vital and less productive, and will be sending its precious life resources toward a growth that isn't serving the whole of the tree.

Proper pruning is an art. It requires a great deal of awareness and finesse to know what to cut, how to cut, and what to leave to ensure that the tree flourishes and produces bountiful fruit of exquisite and delicious quality. When you remove what is not serving the vitality of the whole, you allow for the fullness of the natural, organic blossoming to happen. This is an allowing, not a forcing. You simply are supporting what innately wants to happen.

Aligning with your "yes!" requires learning the art of pruning your life. Is your life feeling crowded? Do you have a sense that you are investing your life-energy where you are not getting returns?

Just as with a fruit tree, pruning your life needs to happen on a regular basis. As the one who is uniquely responsible for tending to your own vitality, you are the only one who can learn the subtle art of pruning your life.

So what might it be time for you to let go of, to prune away? What no longer belongs in your life? What might you need to shed? What clutter might you need to clear away to free up your life-energy to be fully devoted to what you have to give in life, and what you are here to receive? In other words, what is your life-energy currently feeding that is not in alignment with your "yes!"?

This is about unleashing your vitality and releasing the energy that is caught in the heaviness and entanglement of what no longer belongs. Pruning needs to happen in every dimension of your life. Sometimes it just takes a little snip of a tiny twig, and sometimes it requires getting the saw out to remove a large branch that is heading in an unhealthy direction or blocking the light from the branches that feel juicy and full of life goodness for you.

So, where do you get started with the pruning? Wherever is most obvious, and you might start small until you get the hang of it. Below are some examples of places you might begin pruning your life. Grab your journal now and as you read through each of the categories, pause before going onto the next and do some stream-of-consciousness writing. What might there be for you to prune in that aspect of your life to allow the new emergent growth to thrive? When you finish reading through all of them, you might want to take some time to see if there are any other things that you see to prune in your life that might not have been captured in the examples below. Trust whatever comes, and remember that you don't need to prune everything all at once. In fact, overpruning a tree can create instability in its new growth, and the same can be true for you.

PHYSICAL BELONGINGS: You might take a look around at your material possessions and see what belongs and what doesn't belong at this point in your life. Do you have clothes that you never wear? Might there be things that you own that you never use, that could use an upgrade, or that somehow don't represent who you are now, or the person you are becoming? I can't tell you how empowering it can be to lighten your load and make room for physical belongings that do align with who you are now.

HOUSEHOLD CLUTTER: It is amazing how much life-energy can be trapped in the physical clutter around your house, desk, car, or work. Clutter can feed into the same inefficiencies and mental distraction that we discussed around multitasking in the last chapter. You can't really ignore clutter completely. It does impact you. And the freedom, lightness, and energy that come from taking a whole bunch of stuff to Goodwill, recycling it, or organizing it for future use can be profound. In a way this is like facing and embracing your shadows in a physical form.

A groundbreaking social study done by UCLA researchers and shared in the book *Life at Home in the Twenty-First Century: 32 Families Open Their Doors* examined the relationship between the home environment and health. The researchers discuss how their work with families is showing that "for the first time, we can link measurably high densities of household objects—what we call 'stressful' house environments—with physiological responses that can markedly compromise homeowner health. That is, conspicuous consumption and constant clutter (as defined and experienced by the residents themselves) may be affecting some mothers' long-term well-being. Cortisol data indicate that fathers are relatively unaffected by the mess."[57] It's interesting to note the gender difference that was revealed in this study, which might offer insight into your own experience in your home, whether you are a man or a woman.

Laura, whom I mentioned earlier, found this practice of decluttering to be surprisingly transformative. "Decluttering was working for me on multiple levels," she said. "It served as a metaphorical entry to the process of bringing things up and letting them go. Decluttering is about making space for new things in my life, making space for new vitality. When I go through my things and pack them up, I always have a moment of relief and release. And I never think back on what was in those bags once they are gone. The impact on my life has been to deepen my willingness to let go. Letting go of things on the concrete physical level has opened me up to letting go on the emotional level. Now, I regularly look at what's not working in every area of my life—with friendships, with activities, with everything. I ask myself, 'Do I need it?'"

VOLUNTEER COMMITMENTS: What have you said "yes" to that really wasn't a true "yes!"? Perhaps you did so out of a sense of obligation, duty, or habit? Perhaps you didn't want to disappoint someone? This is ripe terrain to explore your shadows around what may motivate you to accumulate commitments that aren't inspiring and life-giving to you. There are an abundance of ways in which we can serve and offer our gifts in life, and it doesn't serve anyone if you are feeding your life-energy into acts of service that don't give you returns. Let them go, and listen for the clear "yes!" when you commit to things in the future.

RELATIONSHIPS: This is a big one, and can be very tender territory. Whether it's a work colleague, an old friend, a family member, a new social group you are a part of, someone you are dating, or your spouse, relationships are ripe territory to assess for pruning. As humans, we are social creatures and need connection and intimacy of all kinds in order to be nourished in our aliveness. Yet if we are not being discerning for ourselves about who we are investing our life-energy with, relationships can also be an enormous source of *dis*-ease and suppressed vitality.

In a very telling study, researchers looked at how marital-stress levels influence how quickly a wound will heal. Forty-two married couples of varying ages were brought to a hospital where they were given a few small blister wounds on two separate occasions. The first time they were guided in discussions with one another around social support, and the second time they discussed a marital disagreement. The researchers monitored the healing of the wounds both times and found in their statistical analysis of the results that the wounds healed more slowly after the conflict discussions, and that those couples who demonstrated higher levels of hostility across both interactions took almost twice as long to heal as the couples who showed low hostility. The correlating increase in pro-inflammatory cytokines, or proteins, seen alongside the slower wound healing amplifies the take-home message from the study: that relationship stress most definitely negatively impacts health and physiological well-being and can contribute to an accelerated occurrence of a number of diseases.[58]

Of course, relationships are not an easy thing to simply prune, especially our more intimate ones. But acknowledging their influence on our well-being is a critical first step in being willing to take action.

In his book *Vital Friends: The People You Can't Afford to Live Without*, researcher Tom Rath shares some of his data regarding the influence of our social circles:

> I asked a group of 104 colleagues to respond to a brief questionnaire about their own diet and their best friend's diet. It turned out the two were even more closely intertwined than I would have guessed. Those who reported having a best friend with a "very healthy" diet were more than five times as likely to have a very healthy diet themselves, when compared to people who had best friends with an average diet. When I asked a similar question about "your best friend's level of physical activ-

ity," the results were just as striking. In fact, of the 104 people surveyed, among those who had a best friend who was *not* physically active, *not one* was very physically active themselves.[59]

These same results were corroborated later in a random study of 1,005 people.

Sometimes it is a matter of shifting how you relate, sometimes it is how much you relate, and sometimes a stronger boundary needs to come into place that effectively prunes a person completely from your life. This is complex territory and I would encourage you to get some personalized support if you are exploring changing the terms of how you relate with someone significant in your life.

WORK: Whether you work part time, full time, more than full time, or are not working but yearn to, this realm of your life has a huge impact on your state of vitality. We each have a different relationship with our work. For some it is about following their life's calling, the expression of their gifts. For others it is more of a means of supporting the lifestyle they enjoy. Wherever you may fall on the spectrum, the reality is that a great deal of your life-energy is invested in the work you do each day. Are you getting returns on that investment? How so? What's the impact on your life-energy? Are you enlivened by your work, or do you feel exhausted simply thinking about it? Most of us will work 100,000 hours before we retire, so the impact on our lives cannot help but be significant. In considering whether you might need to prune this part of your life, ask yourself if it is more about renegotiating the terms of your work—the schedule, hours, type of work, vacation time, etc.—or is it about letting that job go and creating or finding work that will be more fully aligned with your "yes!"?

HOME: Is the place that you are living feeding you? How might your home not be fully supporting your sense of vitality and aliveness? You might assess the physical location, as well as the design of the home. What might you be able to change in the arrangement and layout of your home that could better support you? Would pruning your home actually lead you to moving to another location? Might you thrive if you were living in the heart of the city instead of out in the suburbs or a small town? Or perhaps you know deep down that you need to be out in nature every day, and your current home simply doesn't offer you that. Is your home too big for your needs, and taking unnecessary time and energy to maintain? Or do you need more space to be able to creatively flower? Whatever your preferences and unique needs may be, your home needs to be a haven for you, a place for you to recharge, restore, let down, and be held in deep nourishment. If it is not that now, see if you can explore what would transform it.

BELIEFS: It is astounding how significantly our beliefs can shape our lives. We touched on this in Key #2: Facing and Embracing Your Shadows, and much of the work of pruning unconscious beliefs, perspectives, and paradigms falls within that realm of shadow work. This includes stories you have about yourself, your capacities, and who you are or could be. When you shed the ideas of who you are supposed to be, it allows you to come into an authentic relationship with yourself. You will not be able to discern what alignment feels like until you do this. All of these beliefs can be like cages you unknowingly stay inside of. As you think about pruning your life, it's a good opportunity to revisit your beliefs. By letting go of beliefs that no longer serve us, we can free up an enormous amount of space in our lives. And not only do we open up space, but we also free ourselves to have the energy, perspective, and outlook to more easefully follow through with the things we know bring us alive.

CLEARING INTERNAL SPACE: This is a more subtle category of pruning, yet one that is vital. Your body may be holding onto emotions from your past, without you even realizing it. The tensions and traumas that we go through ripple out into every aspect of ourselves—physically, mentally, emotionally, and spiritually. If these emotions get stored in the body, they take up critical energy and internal space and can contribute to ongoing health challenges. When you go through a difficult experience, you may initially be aware of the emotions. You cry, get angry, or feel afraid. You may even notice a physical correlation. A backache or migraine that comes on with stress. But you may not be aware of the ongoing connection between your emotions and your body. Sometimes those experiences move through quickly and sometimes they linger within us, for days, weeks, or many, many years.

What are you holding onto in your physical body, your emotions? How have you become attached to your daily tensions and the ways your posture, muscles, breath, and emotional bracing almost protect and guard those parts of yourself? What about the traumas in your past? How are you still identifying with and holding them physically, emotionally, and spiritually in your body-home? This area of pruning is multilayered and intimately linked with your shadows (Key #2). It's common to need professional and social support when you are engaged with this work. There are so many ways, both with and without professional support, to release, move, and prune on these levels through various psycho-emotional-somatic pathways. You might try somatic therapies, dance, vocalization, journaling, sexual release, and emoting to help clear energy from the body and mind. The main thing is to incorporate this kind of clearing regularly into your life, to see how you can open the pathways to release before these emotions become deeply rooted and crystallized into your sense of self.

As all of these examples show, saying an authentic "no" is an act of saying "yes!" to your life-energy. Remember, no one but you can tend to your life-energy and vitality, so it is your responsibility to be discerning about what you are saying "yes" to. If you are someone who habitually says "yes" and then regrets it later, something you can try as a way to strengthen your "no" muscle is to simply respond to every request with, "I'll need to think about it, and get back to you." This will give you time to fully consider the prospect. This can work between you and yourself too if you tend to get easily excited and drawn in a lot of directions. Pause and tell yourself that you won't make a decision until tomorrow (or next week). Let it percolate so that you can learn the art of greater self-discernment. Take some time to tune in to what your truth is, and listen for that guidance as to whether this is where your life-energy is wanting to be shared. With time, after you give yourself that buffer of response, you will get better and better at being clear and honest with yourself in the moment of a request and responding accordingly. But until then, there is nothing wrong (and a lot right!) about gifting yourself the time to reflect and get clear.

The most important part of pruning is to practice self-honesty and trust. When we have the courage to prune away something significant, we can't know what will be given the opportunity to grow and blossom as a result, or where it will lead us in our lives. One really pivotal example of this in my own life happened after three-and-a-half years of my five-year naturopathic medicine doctoral program. I woke up one day as I was studying for finals and confronted myself with the acknowledgment that I was completely burned-out with school. I had lost touch with why I was there, with what that education was about for me. I was going through the motions, jumping through the hoops with the end goal in sight, but not appreciating the journey.

I realized that morning that I didn't have to live that way. And so I went into school the next day and filled out a form to take a leave of absence, starting that next quarter. That break ended up being two years, and included a round-the-world journey that was very much akin to a modern-day pilgrimage.

During that time, I let go of everything: who I thought I was, what I thought I was supposed to be doing, where I thought I was meant to be. It was a stripping away, a groundlessness, and it was scary, intense, disorienting, and so very alive. I felt like I was connecting with my authenticity at a level that I never had. I was free, and not just in the sense that I didn't have a structured flow to my day or a place I needed to be. I felt free within, like I had broken out of some cage that I didn't know had been there. I began to relax into myself, my body, and who I was at a level that I had never known. And looking back, that was just the beginning.

I was coming into contact with the true heart of the medicine that I was here to bring forth. While informed by my naturopathic training, the healing I had to offer was actually connected to this deeper ground of life that I was coming to know. Interestingly, during those two years, I wasn't taking lots of supplements or going to the many health practitioners I had been seeing, and yet I was coming alive again, perhaps more so than I had ever been. This did not go unnoticed by me. My exploring, curious mind was still keeping tabs. There was something I was learning at a cellular level that was part of what I am here to bring to the world.

I'm not suggesting that everyone should take two years to nomadically explore the world. But I do recommend that we each take a deep inward journey like the one I took during those years. It became a journey about letting go of what I didn't need anymore, reprioritizing what was truly important in my life, caring for myself, and listening to the feedback from my body-home. It led to a feeling of generosity and spaciousness within myself.

When I returned to my graduate studies after those two years and navigated the hallways of that school, my former classmates would walk right by me, or would walk by and do a double take. And I knew it wasn't just because of my long hair. I looked different. I felt different. I had been through a true metamorphosis and it was like I had cellularly changed.

I have no doubt that I would not be able to offer all that I do for my clients, nor would I have been able to write this book, if it were not for that sabbatical. What grew forth from that pruning is so deeply connected with the heart of my life, with the essence of who I am here to be, with my "yes!"

Whether you go through a major pruning, like I did, or you simply trim away a few unnecessary twigs, you'll find that when you integrate the art of saying "no" in a way that aligns with your "yes!," your life begins to feel more spacious. Virtually all of my clients come to me with a sense of being overwhelmed, not having enough time, and feeling like they are so busy it is challenging to carve out the space to care for themselves. Aligning with your "yes!" allows you to create space in your life. Room to breathe. Room to let down. To hold yourself. To be held. To play more, rest more, sleep more, love more. You no longer need to live in self-denial.

And when you begin living with more spaciousness, there is now room to consciously invite in what truly aligns with your "yes!" When you let go, you become receptive to what belongs in your life *now*, what is intimately yours to be, have, and do. Your unique purpose. Your life's calling. What nourishes you in such a way that you shine from the inside out. When you are open and inviting to all of these wonderful revelations, you will glow and effortlessly bring to life what is yours to bring to life. Gratitude for being alive and having the opportunity to express your uniqueness is woven into how you move through your days. You consciously create and author your life by editing out what doesn't belong, and inviting in what does. As Robert Louis Stevenson says, "To know what you prefer, instead of humbly saying Amen to what the world tells you you ought to prefer, is to have kept your soul alive."[60]

You can only start the journey from where you are at now. Turn on that inner GPS system and begin in the way only you can.

EXPERIMENTING WITH PLAYFUL CURIOSITY

"At the height of laughter, the universe is flung into a kaleidoscope of new possibilities."
—JEAN HOUSTON

WHEN WAS THE last time you played? I hope it wasn't somewhere in the long-forgotten recesses of your childhood. Play is an essential part of adult life, just as it is essential in the life of the child. Yet too many adults don't make time for play in their lives.

This key is about bringing play back into your life and into your relationship with health and self-care. I call it Experimenting with Playful Curiosity. I love this key because it frees us from the risk of health and self-care becoming a burden or too serious. It releases us from all of the rights and wrongs. It gets us out of perpetuating the boom-and-bust cycle of frustration, failure, and shame. In working with this key, you get to let go of the rulebook! You get to release yourself from what you think you are "supposed to be" doing, and instead do what you *want* to do. You no longer need to grip so tightly to the activity of managing yourself. In other words, this key guides you to heal your relationship with health.

If you are like most of the adults I work with, the idea of prioritizing play in your life can be one of the more challenging aspects of the path toward vitality. It may even feel foreign, like you need to relearn what it is to play. It can help to access a childhood memory of when you were playing in a carefree, innocent, unselfconscious way. See if you can recall in your body how it felt to play in that way. What feelings arise? What does it evoke for you?

For me, play evokes freedom, lightness, laughter, and creativity. Of course, as adults, we can layer on all sorts of competitive energy and put too much focus on winning. Yet pure play is completely free of these elements. Pure play isn't about winning; it is about the joy of experiencing an openhearted, silly, carefree, uninhibited creative energy flow through you. There isn't an attachment to a particular outcome. You simply experiment, try things out, see what happens. You follow your curiosity, open yourself to the experience of it all, have fun, and enjoy the process. Innocent child play moves naturally toward what feels good, to what makes you feel alive and evokes your sense of "yes!"

In today's world, most adults feel the unshakeable weight of responsibility. We need to be productive, get things done, take care of others, and show up to help save the world. There is a seriousness that pervades our adult culture, and even our outlets for downtime typically don't evoke the free spirit of play. This serious orientation is most certainly brought to how we approach our self-care—there tends to be nothing playful or fun about it. That weight of responsibility gets us all twisted up in confusing patterns of strictness toward ourselves followed by rebellion and avoidance. We find it difficult to let go of the feeling that there is something we ought to be doing that we aren't, to let go of the resulting guilt.

Yet play is essential for adults, and I believe it is essential for our health and well-being. As a recent NPR report concluded, "Playtime doesn't end when we grow up. Adults need recess too."[61] Dr. Stuart Brown, founder of the National Institute for Play, writes, "I have found that remembering what play is all about and making it part of our daily lives are probably the most important factors in being a fulfilled human being."[62]

If you're still thinking that this sounds too frivolous for something as serious as your health, consider that vast amounts of research have now been done to prove the importance of play. As Brown writes, "Neuroscientists, developmental biologists, psychologists, social scientists, and researchers from every point of the scientific compass now know that play is a profound biological process. It has evolved over eons in many animal species to promote survival. . . . In higher animals, it fosters empathy and makes possible complex social groups. For us, play lies at the core of creativity and innovation."[63] And he goes a step further: "I don't think it is too much to say that play can save your life. It has certainly salvaged mine. . . . Play is the vital essence of life. It is what makes life lively."[64]

What if you could bring an orientation of play to how you care for yourself, and how you move through your life? If you're reading this book, chances are that you're feeling in some way stuck or frustrated in relationship to your health and self-care. So isn't it time for some creativity and innovation? And what better tool to use than the one evolution designed for just that purpose? As Brown writes, "The genius of play is that, in playing, we create imaginative new cognitive combinations. And in creating those novel combinations, we find what works."[65] Key #6 is all about experimenting imaginatively with your own life, in a spirit of playful curiosity, and finding out what works for you.

A MORE FEMININE APPROACH

As I've said, most adults I meet take an overly serious approach to their own health, but one of the most extreme cases I ever worked with was that of Rachel, a forty-six-year-old editor in Seattle. And it was hardly surprising. She had been navigating chronic illness her entire life. She'd been diagnosed with diabetes when she was six years old and had multiple hospitalizations as a kid. Once, she had even been in a coma for a week. She seemed to fall prey to one infection after the next.

As an adult, she had a long list of diagnoses in addition to the diabetes, including rheumatoid arthritis (chronic pain), chronic fatigue, irritable bowel syndrome, sore throats, and strange rashes. When she began working with me, her job as an editor kept her under the pressure of tight deadlines, which she had no control over; at times she felt like she was working 24/7. It was no surprise that her stress level was high.

When I asked her about her health journey, she told me, "After I was diagnosed with the diabetes, my parents got a postage scale, and they used to weigh whatever I was going to eat. I could only eat things that were on the diet plan from the nutritionist, and only at the designated times and in the designated amounts. I had to test the sugar in my urine several times each day, and have insulin injections at least once or twice each day. I was often sick and on antibiotics, and I still periodically wound up in the hospital. I think I was tremendously angry about not being able to just live like a regular kid. Then the last time I was hospitalized, when I wound up in a coma for a week, I was very angry that I wasn't just allowed to die. I felt betrayed by my parents and by my own body."

She paused, the pain and anger of all those years shadowing her face. "I don't think I told anyone how I felt."

Rachel's harrowing story was one of feeling powerless and out of control. Her parents and her doctors dictated everything she did as a child. And even though she's now a grown adult, she still feels like she has no freedom, because that spirit of control has taken root in her mind and body. She weighs every decision obsessively in terms of how it is going to affect her health.

"You know," she said, with a wry smile, "at one point in my life I lived on the streets for a while to see what it was like . . . and it was one of the happiest times of my life."

This key, Experimenting with Playful Curiosity, has been profoundly liberating for Rachel. "I have lived according to all of these crazy rules to make myself feel safe, and all it did was keep me tense, stressed, and with a lot of anxiety. Since I'm naturally curious, it's much easier to try something out, with a feeling of 'Let's find out what happens if I do this for a week or two,' rather than having everything feel like a chore that I have to do even though I don't want to. Now, it becomes a choice instead of an obligation. I come alive with experimenting. It feels good."

I asked her how the experimentation had changed her orientation. "At first, my focus was mostly on trying to prevent something bad from happening," she said. "But after a while, I adapted, and the next thing I knew I was no longer focused on avoiding bad things—I started being able to enjoy the good things and focus more on what I want and how to make it happen."

Through her experimentation, Rachel is feeling more relaxed and more creative, and she's finally learning to trust herself, her friends, her family, and her coworkers. She describes the shift as a more feminine approach. "I always did things in a masculine way, going after something external. I wasn't happy with that but I didn't really know anything else. I see now that I had to feel safe enough to let my guard down to be able to find another way."

This feminine approach is something Rachel has enjoyed experimenting with. "I began having nice scents in the house, and nice music in the background and soft fuzzy things to cuddle up with. I kept looking for ways to indulge myself. Through doing this, I recognized that I used to turn to food because that was one of the only ways that I allowed myself comfort, nourishment, and indulgence. As I have other sensual comforts, food is less important and I don't fixate as much on it." Rachel's health is a complex puzzle, and she is still sorting it out, but the shift in her orientation has changed her life dramatically.

RELAXING INTO CURIOSITY

If you think about it, the degree to which most of us assume we can have everything figured out and under control is ridiculous. None of us have any clue what this is all really about! Being alive. Being in a body. Consciousness. The universe. We may have spiritual beliefs, scientific understandings, or an intuitive knowing of something that feels like truth, and yet, when it comes down to it, we can admit that we really don't know. While this may evoke an existential angst, I want to propose something else. Consider how it would be to relax into that place of not knowing, to be at ease with the recognition that so much of our experience on this planet is mysterious.

What does this have to do with your health? Well, it helps to admit that we humans are kind of making it up as we go. What if we were to embrace everything in life, including our health, as a game, as one big ongoing experiment to play in? To experiment means to try something out without being sure of what the outcome will be. It requires an orientation of learning, of curiosity, of interest to see what will happen. And that's a position that is in fact much more in alignment with reality than pretending we have it all under control with our predictions, our theories, and our protocols.

Internationally recognized expert in holistic medicine Bernie Siegel, MD, points out that in embracing this spirit of curiosity, we are actually being more "scientific" than when we think we know how everything works. "When we think we know the truth, we become closed-minded and very *un*scientific," he writes. "A true scientist has no fixed beliefs and so can experiment in the hopes of learning the truth. . . . By keeping that invaluable inner child's perspective as we grow up and go through life, we are assured of remaining open to all possibilities, whatever we are evaluating at any point in our lives. Once we start to self-censor, we are lost."[66]

I'm suggesting that in this scientific spirit of relaxed curiosity, you start to playfully design new experiments with your own life and to be interested in how things unfold. Building on what we've discussed in the previous keys, your experiments can be informed by paying attention to your body and to what brings you alive.

What if change didn't need to be so hard? What if transformation didn't necessarily require so much effort and pain? What if you could simply make a commitment to try something out for a while and see what happens? What if you enter the "experiment" with simple questions in mind: How does it make me feel? Does this increase my aliveness and optimum vitality or does it reduce it?

When I discovered this key, Experimenting with Playful Curiosity, for myself, it felt completely revolutionary. It seemed strange how profound it was, as in a way it seems utterly simple and obvious, and yet it dramatically changed how I approached my self-care and brought such a lightness and ease to my daily life as a result. For that reason, I look forward to introducing this key to my new clients. Almost every time, I get to see a visible sense of relief come over their tired, anxious faces: A baffled smile. A change of posture. A spark in their eyes as they realize they are just creating an experiment, not locking themselves into anything, not beating themselves into submission.

Most of us live in constant fear of failure. When you experiment with playful curiosity, failure isn't an option. You are merely trying things out and seeing what happens. When you relax into framing your choices and intentions as experiments, rather than a habitual "should," you get to be a conscious explorer of yourself, heeding the feedback you receive. You are released from the cage of needing to get it right, or being afraid that you made the wrong choice. All of the feedback you receive is simply data to guide you in designing your next experiment. Nothing ever stops. You stay in motion.

THE EXPECTATION TRAP

One of the traps that I see most of us fall into on our health journeys is getting stuck with unhelpful ideas like, "I need to stick to _____ in order to be healthy," or "If only I _____, then I'd be healthy." In your journal, see if you can fill in the blank for each of those sentences right now. Don't think about it too much or edit yourself. Simply see what is there in your consciousness. Let yourself be surprised.

Here are some common responses I've seen from participants in my workshops:

+ "I need to stick to a regime of going to the gym five times a week in order to be healthy."

+ "I need to stick to my diet and stop eating ice cream in order to be healthy."

+ "I need to lose 40 pounds in order to be healthy."

+ "I need to go to bed by 10:00 p.m. in order to be healthy."

Obviously, we all have our own versions of these statements. When you look at yours, how do they feel to you? Are you living up to your own expectations? Because that's what these are. Expectations. Ideals we compare ourselves to, and judge ourselves against. Are we "doing it right" or are we "doing it wrong"? These statements are, more often than not, absolute statements, lines drawn in the sand between what we consider to be "success" and what we consider to be "failure." I'm sure you know which side of that line you tend to find yourself on.

Here's the thing: You are complex and nuanced. And you are constantly changing, growing, and evolving. The contexts in your life are always changing—your jobs, relationships, homes, passions. Think back to fifteen years ago. Who were you then? What was different about your life, preferences, and priorities? Quite a lot, I imagine!

Your orientation to self-care needs to be allowed to evolve and move with you; otherwise you are setting yourself up for entering a never-ending cycle of failure, self-judgment, and shame. There is nothing linear or static in a vital life. All you need to do is look out in nature to see how true and undeniable this is. Life is always evolving. In her book *Maps to Ecstasy*, Gabrielle Roth writes, "Disease is inertia. Healing is movement. If you put the body in motion, you will change."[67]

Just as a gardener tries out what she thinks will best support her plants, monitoring them carefully to see how they respond, so you can garden yourself in the same way: if you aren't thriving in the way you want to be, you can experiment with different strategies for nourishment and support. A good gardener knows that when you are tending life, there is no prescription that works every time. The environment is always changing—weather patterns, the mineral content in the soil, the health of the fungi and bacteria that add vital nutrients and influence the way in which the earth drains or holds water. Add to that the diversity of the seeds and the uniqueness of how each plant responds, and you can see that no matter how much science has advanced in large-scale agriculture there are ongoing challenges that make gardening and farming far from an exact science.

You, too, are dynamic and move in a constantly changing ecosystem of your own life circumstances, relationships, and priorities. Take the advice of Eckhart Tolle, author of *The Power of Now*: "Give up defining yourself—to yourself or to others. You won't die. You will come to life."[68] By embracing an orientation of experimentation, you are able to honor and celebrate your evolution. You are able to easefully adapt and be flexible. You are able to dance with life, creatively and playfully. And the freedom you experience in this will play a huge role in your healing.

DESIGN YOUR FIRST EXPERIMENT

So let's explore what this all might look like in your life. What is something that you would like to find a creative new relationship to? Choose something concrete. Is it an aspect of a relationship, a physical issue, something work- or service-oriented, a behavior, or a habit? For example, one client, David, created an experiment of turning off all technologies at 8:00 p.m. each night. Another client, Alyssa, created an experiment to declutter her house.

Begin to formulate one experiment that you'd like to create and engage with for the next two weeks in relationship to whatever you've chosen. Just two weeks. A commitment of that length is totally reasonable, right? It's long enough that you get to really feel the pattern change of your experiment and how it affects the way in which you experience life and how you feel in your body. But it's short enough that even if the experiment has discomforts associated with it, you can see the end. Make sure when you plan your experiment to get very concrete and detailed about when, how, what, who. Your experiment needs to be grounded in the realities of your daily life.

Here are some criteria you can use when planning your experiment. It should be:

+ Something that feels fun, nourishing, and unique to you. Try not to frame it only in terms of deprivation, something you have to "give up" (instead, consider the benefits or opportunities you're giving yourself).

+ Something you haven't tried before.

+ Simple and realistic. When some of my clients initially design their first experiment it seems like they've rolled ten different experiments into one. Try to keep it singular, simple, and doable, so that you can begin to disentangle yourself from the boom-and-bust, burnout cycle. You have a lifetime to explore, after all!

+ Consider it an added bonus if you are able to meet multiple needs and forms of nourishment in one experimental design (i.e., you might sign up for a ten-week cooking class with a friend, with the intention to try out the recipes at least once a week at home. In addition to the social connection with your friend and the built-in support for creating healthy, nutritious meals on a regular basis, you are learning new skills for nourishing yourself and others).

David's experiment with turning off the technology each night opened up space for him to have more intimate time connecting with his partner, and time to do things like take a bath, read, and relax before bed. He found that he began going to sleep earlier and waking more rested than he had in years.

Alyssa had been overwhelmed by the clutter in her house for a long time. She worked full time and had two energetic daughters and a busy husband. She decided to create an experiment that included committing to two fifteen-minute decluttering sessions per week. She would turn some dance music on, dance for a couple of minutes or so, then dive into the decluttering project of her choice. She found that it was so satisfying for her, and strangely fun, that she ended up usually spending longer than the fifteen minutes she originally challenged herself to. Alyssa is amazed with how much energy has been freed up in other areas of her life since she has been able to create space and order in her home.

This kind of experiment is like a low-risk investment. You're not putting your entire life savings, or life-energy in this case, on the line. You are investing for two weeks. And if you like the returns, you can choose to invest in the same way for another two weeks. Or if you don't like what you get back, you can invest in something else. Overall, you will get far better results with this approach than with a high-risk one—you are able to invest yourself fully, yet with almost no risk. I can't imagine a more fruitful way to reap the returns of increased vitality in your life.

ACTIVE LEARNING

An essential thing to remember is that you are not going for a linear outcome. You are *playing*, with all the nuance and unpredictability that playing implies. Everything you are engaging with is part of the experiment. If you set an intention for two weeks and it lasts two days, that's feedback and an impetus to begin the next experiment.

The wonderful thing about this orientation of experimentation and playful curiosity is that you set yourself up to be actively learning. So if you make choices that run your energy into the ground, you get to be present with what happened, learn from it, and have that learning inform how you approach your next experiment. We let children fall and pick themselves up—we, too, need to apply that principle to ourselves.

Now would be a great time to connect back with your inner Mama Bear. If she saw you stumble and find your balance again, she'd smile, knowing you are cultivating your awareness and your core strengths. If you tripped and fell on your face, she'd go to you, maybe wait to see if you are able to stand back up on your own, and help you if needed. Either way she'd wrap you in a sweet, loving hug, letting you know that you are okay. And she would appreciate that you are learning ways to have more discernment and consciousness as you move through your new life. It's natural to feel pain, and to have discomfort. In fact, without these, life would feel numb and unreal. We haven't failed when we experience these things, we are simply experiencing the fullness of life.

CHECKING IN: *Pause for a moment here in your reading and let all of this sink in. Be present in your body, feeling all the subtle signals letting you know you are alive. Tune into your emotional state in the moment and how you access that in your body. And let yourself open in this moment in the spirit of playful curiosity to see what might be arising for you—new insights, new wonderings, another experiment to play with?*

FREE YOUR WILD!

As we experiment with playful curiosity, we dance with the creative emergence of life. We don't need to think of ourselves as problems that need to be fixed, assuming there is something fundamentally wrong about us. We can step back and take the bigger view of the process and explore with curiosity how we can best support ourselves in the midst of our transformation. We can relax into the natural paradox and complexity, not needing to try to fit our lives into a tidy box, or cage, when we are in fact wild and need to be free in order to thrive.

Your vitality knows that you are a wild creature, even if human culture tells you otherwise. I'm sure you have accessed your own wildness in your life—dancing with abandon, exploring the sublime beauty of the wilderness, or feeling your primal nature break free during sexual engagement. These moments tell us unequivocally that we are gloriously vital and alive! Key #6 is a way to weave your wildness into your daily life by acknowledging fully that you can't be tamed and boxed in. You need to honor your ever-changing self that wants and needs to express itself and explore in new ways. Your way of caring for yourself must embrace this fluidity and emergence, the complexity, nuance, and paradox.

As Jungian analyst Clarissa Pinkola Estés writes in her classic book *Women Who Run With the Wolves,* "The wild nature pours out endless possibilities, acts as a birth channel, invigorates, slakes thirst, satiates our hunger for the deep and wild life. Ideally, this creative river has no dams on it, no diversions, and no misuse."[69]

Let yourself feel the freedom and release that comes from unleashing your inner wildness and all the possibilities it brings with it. In those moments when you would habitually fall into shame, give up, or get stuck in what you think of as failure, remind yourself that you are always in motion, and that you can start where you are, and try the next thing. This is how life becomes play—when we live in our evolution, consciously experimenting, shifting direction, trying on new ways of being, sticking with those that work for us, until they no longer do, then letting them go. Embracing change is part of our intimate dance with this great mystery of which we are a part.

Life is much more fun when we let go of our tight hold on who we think we are supposed to be and what we think we are supposed to be doing. You may remember how the combination of Key #3: Strengthening Your Self-Awareness Muscles and Key #4: Cultivating Resilience allows you to own that you are your own best health guide. Key #6: Experimenting with Playful Curiosity supports you in taking it one step further. When you read books on health, or a popular blog, or a friend tells you about the next best thing they have tried, you can take in the recommendations, theories, and knowledge of others and try them on as experiments. You get to see how they make *you* feel, and whether they fit into the realities of your unique flow and dance in life.

The pathway to optimum vitality really isn't what most of us think. Pop out of the box with me here. Love and nurture yourself in these ways, not because you are supposed to, but because when you wake up to the preciousness of life, there's really nothing else that makes any sense whatsoever to prioritize above that. Bring yourself alive. Play in this mysterious game of life. Experiment, try things out, live on the edge—*your* edge. Step into the unknown, consciously stretch yourself, try on new ways of being, new ways of seeing, new ways of knowing. And recognize that in embracing this playful, curious, experimental way of holding yourself in life, you are gifting us all with a fuller, deeper, more authentic expression of you in the world. Your wild, natural self!

CELEBRATING EACH STEP

When you are engaged with this key, you can celebrate each and every step. You can feel the aliveness in staying in motion, in remaining engaged with your process. Eventually, this celebratory attitude becomes a way of life. And you'll see that over time you become more and more skillful at navigating experiments, and more and more discerning and empowered in how you design them and how you live them. You won't get caught in a boom-and-bust cycle on your self-care journey because you will no longer be attached to the journey looking a certain way. If something doesn't work for you, you can explore one of the remaining endless possibilities that may bring you to a place of thriving. The only limit is your own creativity, and that's boundless!

Celebration is innately part of this process, and it's important. You are celebrating each of the little steps that continue to open you into greater freedom, ease, and thriving. You aren't fixated on an end goal that has to be "just so." You are steering your life and responding to what emerges with the spirit of adaptability and flexibility. You are no longer the victim of your circumstances. You expect the unexpected. And because you are experimenting, you won't get derailed as you might have before, because whatever you experience is simply the data to inform you about what to try next.

Being on your health and self-care journey doesn't have to be difficult. While it can certainly be challenging, it can be playful, too. By bringing a sense of humor and flexibility to the journey as well as allowing yourself to feel the pleasure that comes from advocating for your own self-care, your health pilgrimage can be a truly joyful experience. And what could be greater cause for celebration than that?

KEY #7

DISCOVERING
EASEFUL DISCIPLINE

*"There is no freedom without discipline,
no vision without a form."*
—DAVID ALLEN

"I KNEW IT! All of that fun, playful curiosity and experimentation stuff was too good to be true!"

This is often the response I get from clients when I transition from Key #6 to Key #7 and they see the dreaded D-word. *Discipline.* Yes, this one is even more of a trigger than "responsibility." For most of us, it immediately raises the specter of all those "shoulds" that we've struggled with forever, and the sense of inevitable failure and shame that accompanies them.

I wish I could spare you that experience, and tell you that discipline has no place in this journey. But I'd be lying. There is a need for discipline on the road to health and vitality. However, it may not be the kind of discipline you imagine. For starters, it's not in any way at odds with the last key, Experimenting with Playful Curiosity. Not at all! They are like intimate friends, leaning into each other for the support they need to bring you the results you need.

The kind of discipline this key introduces is *easeful* discipline. And as much as that might sound like a contradiction in terms, it's not. As author and public speaker Charles Eisenstein so eloquently says, "True discipline is really just self-remembering; no forcing or fighting is necessary. When used in this way—to remember oneself, to come back into alignment—willpower is natural and energizing, whereas when we are fighting ourselves, it is an ordeal."[70] Before I reveal the new territory, however, it feels important to unpack and see with clear eyes what your relationship with discipline has been like. That way, we can root out any shadow issues that might otherwise subvert your ability to embrace this key.

As I'm sure you've seen in this book so far, while we are talking specifically about health and self-care, the reality is that we are talking about how you are showing up in all aspects of your life. Each of these keys applies to how you engage in your relationships, in your work, as a parent, and as a citizen of your community, country, and world. When it comes to discipline, this certainly continues to be true. Your relationship to discipline ripples out into everything in your life.

Cultural priorities these days focus so much on productivity, efficiency, and getting things done. And most of us are overbusy, overwhelmed, and struggling with the challenges of an information and technology age that never stops demanding more of our time. We're all adjusting and trying to figure out how to make our way in this new reality that is constantly changing. It is taxing on us all, in ways that I think we're only beginning to be able to understand.

Discipline and productivity in our work lives are highly valued, so much so that I find this emphasis creates major obstacles to taking care of ourselves in conscious, nourishing, honoring ways. Therefore, finding easeful discipline in our work lives is as important to our state of vitality as finding easeful discipline around the self-care habit changes we are moving toward. And as we find ourselves shifting these attitudes to our own self-care, we will discover we won't be able to tolerate the old kind of harsh discipline around our work or aspects of our home life. A softening happens, a spaciousness and self-loving that permeates all aspects of our lives. Reframing and disentangling ourselves from cultural priorities and how we take them on can be a huge step toward discovering ease throughout our lives.

As you read this chapter, I invite you to do so with the larger perspective of what you can learn about discipline in all aspects of your life, wherever you may habitually land on the discipline spectrum.

HOW DO YOU TYPICALLY
RELATE TO DISCIPLINE?

CHECKING IN: *Tune in to yourself right now. What happens in your body when you think of discipline? What do you feel, and where do you feel it? What's the emotional quality? What images come to mind when you think about discipline in your daily life?*

Of course, the experience is going to be different for each of us. Yet there are patterns that I've witnessed in my clients, loved ones, and certainly in myself. The topic of discipline can bring out the extremes of where we have gotten so out of balance in our relationship with self-care, and reveal how our quest to be healthy can become so very unhealthy. Here are some of the patterns I've come to see:

Discipline tends to evoke a feeling of contraction and tension—physically, mentally, emotionally, and spiritually. We likely experience a lot of self-judgment around it, with mean, cruel self-talk. We can feel as if we are trying to live up to something that we can't achieve unless we force ourselves into compliance. We tend to think we need to create rigid sets of rules that we then have to live up to, whether or not we may be consciously choosing them in the moment.

In my work with clients, I've found that their relationship to discipline is often correlated with how they relate to self-responsibility. If you think back to our discussion of that in Key #1, there were two inner characters that I pointed to—the Rebellious Teenager and the Strict Parent.

Discipline tends to bump us right up against a pretty contentious internal dynamic between our inner Strict Parent and our inner Rebellious Teenager. The high-handed, strict, parental side of ourselves tells us what to do in no uncertain terms. In order to respond, we rally ourselves to do what we are supposed to be doing, but with absolutely no wiggle room. We can end up relating to ourselves as if we are outside, looking in. This can result in a dissociation that births internal tension, where we are in conflict with ourselves, trying to step up and will ourselves into submission.

Sometimes we obey the inner Strict Parent and feel proud of ourselves for doing so, as if we are doing the right thing and will be rewarded like the good girl or boy we are. And then our Rebellious Teenager takes over, and we resist all the rules. We rebel by stopping the behaviors the Strict Parent mandated, as we are trying to proclaim our autonomy and freedom in life.

My friend and client Sarah, a thirty-year-old yoga teacher, experienced a classic example of this struggle. "I'm a self-motivated, self-disciplined hard worker," she told me, reeling off a long list of her educational and business achievements. "It used to be the case that I could push through anything— pulling all-nighters on a regular basis—and take on more projects than any one person has time in a day to pursue." Sarah initially didn't take much care of her health, skipping meals and depriving herself of sleep. Then, as she became more health conscious, she carried the same strict discipline into that area of her life. "I became somewhat fanatical," she admits, "eating a raw-foods diet, doing intensive cleanses and extended meditation retreats, practicing yoga rigorously. Even when I was feeling sick I'd go to yoga programs, and I actually now have long-standing injuries from this overly ambitious yoga practice." The irony, she reflects, is that "I was doing everything that was wellness oriented to my maximum capacity, and yet I wasn't feeling so well."

Inevitably, at some point she flipped. "I would sometimes have a binge-and-purge effect happen," she admits. "It would all be too much. Everything would fall apart and I would stop all of the practices for a while."

This kind of cycle in relation to discipline can go round and round, back and forth, up and down in every aspect of our adult lives. Does this sound familiar? I don't think I've come across one person who doesn't know this territory intimately, in their own way.

Regardless of where we lie on the spectrum of self-responsibility and discipline, it can feel extremely disempowering, like we are trying to overcome something we assume is fundamentally wrong about who we are inside. We give ourselves over to some idea of what we think we are supposed to be doing and set ourselves up for internal struggle. The entire realm of discipline can be so fraught with this push-pull dynamic. This is the birthplace of our sense of defeat, shame, and failure around being able to create the changes we seek, to step fully into our power and live the thriving life we know we are capable of living. Battling ourselves into submission to be healthy does not lend itself to allowing us to serve ourselves, others, and our collective future with the grace, shining presence, and brilliance that we each innately embody.

I can't tell you how many times I hear clients call themselves "lazy," with the implied self-judgment that they are lacking in discipline. And when I talk about strategies of habit change with some clients I can visibly see their shoulders ride up with the tension coming in as they brace themselves for the self-sacrifice and tight leash that the discipline will entail.

I will tell you what I tell them: *Relax.* The kind of discipline that I'm introducing in this key is not the kind in which we turn toward ourselves with an energetic whip, trying to corral, manage, and control ourselves. We would only treat ourselves with disrespect in that way if we were disconnected from what I introduced in Key #1, the sense of honoring our unique life and living from a conscious awareness of the precious responsibility to steward and care for ourselves. From that orientation, we can shift how we relate to discipline, and it can actually come to feel empowered and generative as it is moving us toward greater aliveness and expression.

This distinction is a tricky thing for many people to grasp. How can we have discipline that isn't forceful and rooted in a heavy-handed will? There's a way to be relaxed and easeful in our discipline, so that we are not only honoring our lives but making an intelligent assessment of what we need to best guide ourselves. We consciously put into place the structures of support that we know will help us to succeed.

Easeful discipline requires you to return repeatedly to your natural vulnerability. As you come into new ways of being you will inevitably shed and let go. While this can be exhilarating, it can also make you feel tender and exposed, like a baby fresh from the womb. Thankfully, your vulnerability is your ally in this key. Your inner Mama Bear energy will be able to scoop you up in a loving embrace and help you to stay in alignment with your commitments, not with rigidity, but with gentle yet fierce determination.

Regardless of where you are on the spectrum of how you relate to discipline, I can imagine that the idea of easeful discipline may seem a bit like wishful thinking. But please give it a chance—I'll be offering you a grounded path to follow that will allow you to discover this for yourself. It is possible!

THE REALITIES OF HABIT CHANGE

With any kind of metamorphosis of growth or healing, we move through transitional periods in which there may be discomfort and disorientation. In reality, it takes time to change longstanding habits, even if we feel we are fully committed. Very few of us can just decide that we're going to create a change and then effortlessly and easefully sustain it without looking back.

In order to create change we do need discipline. We need discipline because we don't always immediately get the positive feedback to tell us that our choices are in alignment with our deep vitality. Have you ever started exercising again after taking a break and found that the first week or two is really uncomfortable? Your muscles ache. It's hard to breathe. You are way more tired than usual. But then you hit a turning point and it doesn't feel so hard anymore. Not only that, but you start to feel really good after you exercise.

Or maybe you have had the experience of eliminating a food from your diet that you suspected wasn't nourishing for you. Those first few days, you might have had all sorts of detox symptoms—cravings for the food, diarrhea, nausea, exhaustion, funny-smelling sweat. And then, later that week or the next, you realize that a lot of your chronic symptoms have eased up, and you feel better.

Detox happens not just physically, but emotionally and psychologically as well. It's similar to the process of a difficult breakup with a partner, when afterward you might confront the urges to call that person every day, and even though it didn't make sense logically, you wanted them to be the one to comfort you through the grief of losing them. We get wired into behavioral and emotional patterns that can be disorienting and hard to change. In the midst of reprogramming, some of the old pathways are still activated, even as we have set ourselves on a different course. If you are only paying attention to the immediate feedback you're getting, and aligning your choices with that, you might be consistently steering yourself back toward choices and behavioral patterns that actually are suppressing your vitality.

We need discipline to help us to move through the discomfort of change. There are times when our symptoms and experience may actually be telling us that it is all way too difficult, and we may actively feel that we don't like what we are doing. We can feel out of balance and disoriented—the ways in which we have previously grounded ourselves in life, the things we once did to feel strong and stable, may not apply anymore, may be shifting and changing. Discipline is what allows us to ride out these often uncomfortable, murky transition times until we get to the feedback that is clearly pointing the way toward our thriving. Because you are, in a sense, reprogramming yourself, and things can feel off-kilter as you are rebooting. All change, on some level, requires a letting go of the old, a dying off, in order to invite in the new. And that's where easeful discipline comes in.

One way to reframe discipline is to acknowledge that we all need structures of support in place to help us through these transitions. Sometimes it takes a while to get the feedback that we are aligning with our "yes!" beneath the superficial *dis*-ease. We have to be willing to face the darkness, discomfort, and disorientation in order to build up the new muscles of awareness and new pathways of integration in our body. This is true whether we are exercising after not having done so for a long time, shifting our diet, rebranding our business, letting go of a relationship, or any other major change we might consider.

Having periods of discipline to help us to move through these difficulties is vital for creating the change that we seek. Yet how can we do so in a way that doesn't become the health-distorting, unhealthy kind of discipline that most of us know all too well?

First, it's important to be informed and honest with yourself about the realities of habit change. Self-help gurus may confidently tell you that it takes twenty-one days, or thirty days, to change a habit, but according to more rigorous research, it takes quite a bit longer than that. A research team at University College London, led by Phillippa Lally, asked 96 people to choose one new habit to try to adopt over a twelve-week period. Participants reported each day on whether or not they did the behavior and how automatic it felt.

The specific habits people chose in the study varied—from drinking a bottle of water daily to taking a fifteen-minute run before dinner. In analyzing the data, researchers wanted to determine how long it took each person to go from starting the new behavior to doing it automatically; in other words, how long it took to become a habit. The answer was, on average, sixty-six days.[71] So be patient with yourself in these times of transition, and be realistic. The good news that the study revealed was that occasionally skipping a day didn't seem to have much impact on the overall success. So don't beat yourself up for not being "perfect."

Habit change is not only a slow process; it's a complex and paradoxical one as well. We humans are complex creatures and for the vast majority of us, we can't just decide we're going to do something and then it happens, at least not beyond a quick fix. To create any real, ongoing change (which is what this book is all about!) we need to engage with three essential components that allow discipline to become easeful.

PUTTING EASEFUL DISCIPLINE INTO PRACTICE

I find that the best way to understand a new process is to actually do it! As
I outline each of the three areas that need to be addressed in order to find
your way to successful, easeful discipline, I invite you to put it to practice
right away. Have your journal on hand as I guide you to

◆ Clarify Your Commitment

◆ Create Strategies

◆ Implement Structures of Support

CLARIFYING COMMITMENTS

You can't have discipline about something until you are really clear about what
it is you are wanting to embrace or do. This brings us back to the designing
of experiments that we discussed in the last key, Experimenting with Playful
Curiosity. Once you're clear about what habit or behavior you want to change
and how, it's time to directly address the realm of commitments. While we
have touched on the topic of deeper life commitments in other chapters of
this book, with discipline they move front and center. Discipline requires
follow-through, and there can't be follow-through without commitment.

In the past, I've related to my commitments with a fierce drive and strict
discipline. Eventually, I ran myself into the ground, dropping into a deep
chronic fatigue that came and went for years. I've emerged on the other side
of that healing and growth to no longer be able to hold that kind of orientation around commitment. What I saw as commitment then was rigid,
single focused, and unconscious to how I was feeling and experiencing my
life as a whole. It was about the achievement ahead, the task to master, the
long list of "shoulds" that I had created for myself to get to where I thought
I needed to be.

What does commitment and dedication look like outside of that strict
approach? Let's start with the intention you set at the beginning of this
book, or the intention that may have evolved as you've been reading. It

might have been to spend more time with the people you love, or to be more connected to nature, or to feel more comfortable in your body, or to have more energy in your daily life. You may have several intentions, but choose one to work with in this chapter.

When we clarify our commitments we take broad intentions and break them down. For instance, if you know that a life priority for you is to feel energetic in your daily life, you might make some specific commitments around your sleep patterns or your rest, play, or work schedule. Or if you know that you come alive when out in nature, you might set some commitments around taking more vacation time, letting go of other commitments, shifting your relationship to work, or simply taking a daily hike. If you intend to spend more time with your family, you might set commitments around shifting the quality of your shared meal times, planning adventures together, or volunteering time at your child's school. It's important to make your commitments specific and doable.

In the next step, you'll break them down further as you strategize how best to achieve them, but it will be easier to strategize if you have already moved from the larger commitment into the more specific areas of focus. Through this process, you will likely come up with at least one initial commitment that will start you off in your exploration of easeful discipline. However, the steps I'll be sharing below in relation to creating strategies and implementing structures of support will often result in new commitments or ideas on how to rework the ones you already have. So after you shed light on the terrain you may naturally circle back to clarifying your commitments in order to set yourself up for a more informed and effective strategy. And of course, as you learned in Experimenting with Playful Curiosity, there is no such thing as right or wrong when it comes to this process. You try something out, and then redesign and try again, learning as you go.

CREATING STRATEGIES

Easeful discipline requires being fiercely honest about all the obstacles, behavior patterns, contexts, people, and so on that trip you up and sabotage you from doing the things that would support you in thriving. And then it requires that you do what it takes to address each and every one—with intelligence, deep compassion and love, and, of course, playful experimentation! Creating strategies allows you to get real about what it will take for you to follow through on your commitments.

Without intelligently looking with clear eyes at the realities of the terrain you are moving into, you will be devoting your life-energy to experiments that have little chance of giving you a return on your investment.

I can't tell you how many times, when I first start working with clients, I hear them name commitments that seem completely unrealistic for what I know of the realities of their daily lives. Jenny, a fifty-two-year-old woman who commutes two hours to a job where she works up to ten hours a day, is exhausted and burned out. She declares that she wants to lose weight and is committed to going to the gym five days a week. She hasn't been going to the gym at all when she sets this intention. When we start to create a strategy, by exploring together when, where, and how this will fit into her daily life, the intention begins to unravel. Not only does she have her commute and work commitments, but she is a wife and mom and it is a priority for her to have time with her family in the evenings. Given that she needs to sleep and rest, there doesn't seem to be any time to go to the gym, let alone go five days a week. Clearly, some more strategizing needs to happen to clarify what would work for her to achieve her commitments. As you can see here too, one intention like wanting to lose weight can reveal a whole lot of territory that can expose the deeper intentions and priorities underneath the initial goal.

Return now to the commitment that you clarified in step one of this process and see if it fits the following description: it's a commitment you've made on your health journey that you have tried to change repeatedly but have struggled in sustaining, and you sense it would make you come more alive if you did it. If so go ahead and use it for the next part of the exercise; if not simply think of a new commitment now that aligns with that description. In other words, choose something that feels authentically like something you would like to do, not something on your list of abstract "shoulds." Now, in your journal, create a stream-of-consciousness list of all of the obstacles that get in the way of you creating this change. Don't overthink, edit, or judge any of these obstacles as silly or irrelevant. Capture everything that comes up for you.

At this stage, you will need to draw on your self-compassion and gentleness: what you may think of as "obstacles" are often very real needs that you have. A perspective that I've found helpful in navigating this territory is that of developmental psychologist Robert Kegan and research director Lisa Laskow Lahey of Harvard University's Graduate School of Education. In their book *How the Way We Talk Can Change the Way We Work*, they explore why it can be so hard to create the changes that we seek. Similar to what we looked at in the second key, Facing and Embracing Your Shadows, these authors ask, "Why do even our sincerest intentions and New Year's Resolutions to clean up our acts have so little power? . . . There may be bigger forces at work, behind the behaviors . . . and if we don't get these forces onto the table they continue to run the show."[72]

Kegan and Lahey go on to describe these forces as "competing commitments": "No matter how hard and genuinely we may work on behalf of our [first] commitment . . . is it possible we are also working—and with more effective results—in service of a competing commitment?"[73] Living in this state of inner contradiction, they explain, creates a "process of dynamic equilibrium that works with breathtaking power and effectiveness to keep things pretty much as they are."[74] Alison, a client who came to me with severe fatigue, was a natural early riser, regardless of when she fell asleep. Needless to say, she felt more rested if she went to bed at 9:30 p.m. Yet she inevitably ended up staying awake until midnight almost every night with her husband. It became clear that she was breaking her commitment to an earlier bedtime because she feared that it would lead to a lack of intimacy and connection with her husband if she did so—this was her competing commitment that won out time and again.

Kegan and Lahey point out that the competing commitment is usually some form of self-protection, or a form of unhappiness that we are trying to avoid. These are not negative or unreasonable things, but their hidden nature makes them tricky. "The problem is not that we are self-protective, but that we are often unaware of being so," write Kegan and Lahey. "Without accepting responsibility for the forms our self-protection takes, we are inclined to view [the competing commitments] as signs of weakness."[75]

Taking responsibility for these competing commitments means recognizing that they may actually be pointing to real needs you have that you need to address, needs that may be calling out for you to consciously align with the "yes!" within so that you can embrace them (remember the fifth key, Aligning with Your "Yes!"). If you are to move forward and free yourself from the "dynamic equilibrium" that Kegan and Lahey discuss, then you will need to find new and creative ways to meet those needs. For Alison,

uncovering the competing commitment that was interfering with her getting the sleep she needed was significant. She shared with her husband her
fear that they might lose intimacy and connection if she went to bed earlier.
As a result, they created new experiments together. They started to set aside
time in the earlier evening and mornings for spending intimate time with
one another so that all of her needs, and his, could be met.

The process of exploring competing commitments may also lead you
back to the second key, Facing and Embracing Your Shadows. Through
this earlier key you can more easily access the roots of the obstacles and the
deeper needs inherent in those competing commitments—it is here where
true breakthroughs can happen. This will not be necessary for every obstacle
that shows up for you, but some of what you discover here will lead you to
some core patterns and beliefs, and perhaps to some unresolved, unhealed
wounds. If you can have the courage to explore what's there, you can guide
yourself toward the freedom, healing, and self-actualization that you seek.

Let's return to the exercise. Now that you've captured your list of obstacles,
turn to a fresh page and mark two columns labeled "Obstacles" and "Strategies." Transfer the obstacles you came up with in your brainstorm to the
first column on this new page, then try to come up with a strategy for each
one, however small or inconsequential it may seem. Some of the obstacles
may require gently and lovingly addressing a real need in the form of a
competing commitment. Other obstacles, however, will be very simple and
straightforward. For example, you may have committed to practice yoga
each morning, but you discover the following obstacles: you don't own a
yoga mat and you have no space to practice. This reveals two important
prerequisites to fulfilling your commitment: buying a yoga mat and clearing some space in your office, for example. Get specific about these kinds
of precursors and set dates to achieve them. If they feel too daunting right
now, perhaps you need to consider starting with a different commitment for
this particular experiment.

As we're wrapping up this section on creating strategies, let's return to
Jenny, who has the intention of losing weight through regular exercise. As
we saw, her current time is so limited with work and family commitments
that going to the gym isn't realistic. So doing an assessment process to create
strategies as we have just discussed is absolutely vital for her success.

We can look to creative ways for her to meet her needs:

1. She could experiment with trying out a bodyweight-based strength-training program that she could do anywhere for just 15 minutes a day, at home or in a break at work. No need to go to the gym, and little impact on her limited time. These programs are highly effective and anyone can do them, at any fitness level.

2. She could also integrate exercise with family time. Going on evening walks with her kids and husband, or going to the park and running around with a Frisbee or a soccer ball would be two ways to do this.

3. Perhaps, in confronting her competing commitments and the real needs that are there underneath the obstacles, Jenny might realize that there is a bigger change wanting to happen. She might come to see that while she might like aspects of her work, the commute, time investment, and stresses aren't allowing her to devote her life-energy to what matters to her most—her family and her sense of vitality. She's tired of feeling tired and is ready to make a bigger change. So a new intention and commitment emerge.

IMPLEMENTING STRUCTURES OF SUPPORT

When you are developing strategies, you will need to consider what kinds of structures will be most supportive for your success. When I use the term "structures," I'm referring to tools, programs, rituals, and more, which I'll be outlining below. What these will provide is a container to relax into. You can trust that there is a process that you've set up to support yourself. When you show up and have your own back and are fully on board to make something happen, you will be able to do what it takes. You're ready to stop beating yourself up for not doing it, and you design the structures that can hold your movement forward. Structures of support keep your awareness and intentions front and center. They are reminders of what you are choosing to truly commit to in life and what your priorities are.

These days, there is no shortage of books, theories, apps, and practices around productivity, self-discipline, and getting things done. Since this is not the main focus of this book, I'll leave it to you to explore the resources out there to find what best supports you. I fully invite you to bring your creativity on board as you design the structures for yourself. And of course you get to experiment with playful curiosity to learn what works best for you.

Here are some ideas to get your creativity jump-started and to help you embrace easeful discipline on your self-care journey:

◆ **Relational Support:** I am a huge proponent of relational support. It is one of the most essential elements for succeeding in creating easeful discipline. In fact, I see it as so foundational that I've dedicated a whole key to it. Key #8 explores in depth how to weave relational support into your discovery of easeful discipline.

◆ **Your Calendar:** Please do not underestimate the power of keeping an intentional calendar. You need to block out the time for those things that don't ordinarily happen, because the reality is you must treat your intentions and experiments as every bit as important as your other commitments—work and family, daily and weekly responsibilities—and schedule them in as if they are appointments with someone else, someone important. Julia Cameron, in her wonderful book *The Artist's Way,* talks of having "artist dates" with yourself to feed your creativity through regular doses of inspiring new experiences and adventure. You can come up with names for your various dates with yourself—na-ture-walk dates, nap dates, dates to sit and journal, yoga-class dates, afternoon-at-the-spa dates, unstructured-play dates, your daily can-dlelit-bath date, or your dates to prepare nourishing food for yourself and your family.

Your scheduling may involve other people, too—date nights with your sweetie on a weekly basis, or getting out with your best friend for a weekly walk. When you schedule things in, and honor them as sacred commitments to yourself, then your experiments get to take root in your daily life.

Sarah, the ultra-disciplined young woman whom I introduced at the beginning of the chapter, came up with a beautiful example of a scheduled support structure. She'd eventually suffered burnout from her "binge-and-purge" cycles, and had been working to create more balance and ease in her life. Engaging with discipline in a new way was a real breakthrough for her. "These days, I have a schedule that intentionally provides focused time for rest and restoration. In adopting easeful discipline, I have come to see that clear commitments and structures need to be there. One thing that I've incorporated more recently as a structure is having Fridays as my 'Source Day'—a day to prioritize some of the things that are foundational to me—time to be in nature, for writing, and for spacious, unstructured, creative dreamtime."

Sarah recalls that, initially, it felt like a big risk to give herself that day, to actually put it in her schedule and cancel everything else. "Yet what I've found," she says, "is that that spacious day feeds everything else that I'm doing."

+ **Programs:** When you are in the new phase of adopting and trying out a new behavior pattern, mindset, or way of being, it can be very helpful to have the structure of a program that someone else has designed. This isn't about deferring your own self-knowing to someone else's expertise; it is about becoming your own health and vitality guide through learning what structures and techniques have worked for others. You can embrace programs as experiments to try out. A program can be found in a book, or these days a plethora of self-guided, home-study programs are available online. Or you can sign up for a locally based program that offers you a protocol, schedule, timeline, etc. Even if you decide after a week that you don't resonate with the approach, you've gotten feedback that can inform an intention and help you experiment with a design that is a better fit for you and the realities of your daily life.

+ **Rituals:** I came to see the power of rituals during my training as a vision-quest guide. Before I had been kind of skeptical, seeing people going through the motions of something that someone else had prescribed for them or that was part of a religious or spiritual tradition. What shifted for me during the vision-quest guide training was that I came to understand the power of self-created rituals; these are rituals that are born from your own creativity and intuition, or from an authentic desire to mark something significant in your life, invite something in consciously, or to evoke a particular state or remembrance for yourself.

I have seen over the years how rituals can be used very effectively inside of the mundane rhythms of our daily life and during times of larger transformation and rebirthing. By consciously creating a ritual for your daily life, you are creating a structure of support for yourself that can help disentangle you from your inner Strict Parent and the harsh disciplinarian that he or she can be. Through ritual, you honor your unique life through an action, a behavior, a mindset, or a pattern you are weaving into your days. For instance, you might have struggled with integrating exercise in your life, trying to will yourself into submission. You could decide that the ritual of a morning walk on the trails near your house starts your day with a spiritual clarity, wakes up your body, gives you time for reflection, and simply feels good! Reframing the walking as a ritual offers you an easy "buy-in" and an easeful discipline.

Rituals can be applied to anything. I know an increasing number of people who are creating a ritual of "no Internet on the weekends" to afford them the ability to slow down, unplug, and focus on what restores them. Or, if you are an entrepreneur who tends to work all the time, you could create a clear ritual, like going out for dinner on Friday nights, that marks the end of your work week, so that you can be sure to shift into a non-business mode for at least one or two days a week. If you are trying to adjust your sleep habits, you might create a nightly ritual of taking an Epsom salt bath with soothing music and candles, to let down from the day and transition into rest.

✦ **Reminders (Love Notes to Yourself!):** Because habit change is as much a mindset shift as a behavior shift, you may find that you benefit from creative ways to remind yourself of your intentions. I like to think of these as love notes to yourself, as you can infuse the reminders with loving encouragement. You can write reminders on Post-it notes, or create image or photo reminders and put them up on your bathroom mirror, at your office desk, or on your bedside table, refrigerator, or front door. Calendar reminders or screensavers that pop up on your phone or computer and gently nudge you toward action can be surprisingly powerful. For example, you could include questions or reminders like, "What do I need right now?"; "How am I feeling in my body in this moment?"; "It's time to stand up and move!"; "Pause, close your eyes, and focus on noticing your breathing for one minute"; or "I get to do my playful experiment now!"

✦ **Inspiration:** Sometimes we lose touch with our priorities and the deeper commitments we have to ourselves. If that happens, the particular experiments or intentions we have can grow flat as they begin to detach from the ground in which they are rooted. Having a library of quotations, inspirational books, audio talks, TED talks, and movies that can serve to gently connect you back to what really matters and what you are deeply committed to can be a vital part of your easeful-discipline journey. If you like audio books, audio classes, or podcasts, you can have them on hand on your smartphone to listen to while you are walking or driving.

✦ **Shaking it Up!:** I have found it vital to shake myself awake when I become stuck in seriousness and rigidity. I personally love having dance parties on a regular basis—by myself or with others. Even if you don't like to dance, find something else that helps you to reactivate the spirit of playfulness and to open your body. Maybe it's a play-date with your dog or cat, giggles with some of your favorite video clips, singing along to some upbeat music you love, or having wild, passionate sex (with yourself or a lover!). Remember to continually come back to loosening and lightening up, to remain flexible and fluid with how you are holding yourself in discipline.

What would you add to this list?

FOLLOW YOUR EASE

If you follow the suggestions in this chapter in the spirit of playful curiosity, easeful discipline will slowly emerge in a particular form that works for you. And it will continue to evolve and change. A discipline that is grounded in what truly brings you alive must inherently be rooted in love and self-nurturing and cannot be rigid and linear in its path. Sarah, the thirty-year-old yoga teacher who prided herself in being hardworking and ultradisciplined, tells me that these days, it is slowly pervading every part of her life. "All those things I did so strictly through the years are things I can use now, but in a different way. When I am practicing any discipline, whether it is a specific dietary practice, meditation, or yoga, I hold it with a lot more spaciousness and forgiveness and a lot more room to play. If I am eating a certain way because my body is feeling better, and I really want a hamburger or a piece of cake, I check in with myself. I don't care so much if it is contrary to a practice that I am exploring. If it feels right, I am just going to enjoy it. I don't do the seesawing with intensity and deprivation anymore so even if I choose something once, it doesn't lead to gluttony. The thing that is emerging for me overall as the essence of easeful discipline is the seeking of pleasure. I look for what feels deeply good and what makes me happy. If I am following that as my guidance, I will do things that challenge me, that are uncomfortable, and that are new, but it will always be from a place of self-nourishment and self-respect instead of pushing myself too hard. And when I do fall into days when I'm pushing too hard, I think to myself, 'What would Dr. Deborah say?' And then I go take a hot salt-water bath and return to my work renewed and with much more easeful discipline."

BRINGING IT ALL TOGETHER

Now that you have had a chance to explore how to bring easeful discipline to your self-care journey (and to your life), I invite you to now connect it with Key #6: Experimenting with Playful Curiosity by creating a fresh new two-week experiment for yourself. Remember to retain that spirit of playful curiosity as you go through the steps:

+ **Clarify the Commitment** you are choosing.

+ **Create Strategies** to ground that commitment in the realities of your daily life in intelligent ways.

+ **Implement Structures of Support** to allow you to relax into a container that is holding you in your experiment.

Try it out, starting today! Play, learn, and be curious with how your experiment nourishes and serves you in your life. Then, apply your learning and try again with a fresh experiment.

INVITING SUPPORT AND CONNECTION

"Life doesn't make any sense without interdependence. We need each other and the sooner we learn that the better for us all."

—Joan Erikson

HERE'S A SOBERING STATISTIC: people with very few social ties are more than twice as likely to die sooner than those with multiple, strong social ties.[76] According to Harvard Medical School, "Dozens of studies have shown that people who have satisfying relationships with family, friends, and their community are happier, have fewer health problems, and live longer," while conversely, "a relative lack of social ties is associated with depression and later-life cognitive decline, as well as with increased risk of mortality."[77] Science seems to have conclusively shown that our circle of relationships is critical for our health and well-being. And yet, if there's one belief I've observed over and over among my clients, it's this: *When it comes to my health and self-care, I'm on my own.*

Many of my clients are men and women who tend to care a great deal for others and who give themselves to improving our world. They give and give and give to their kids, their parents, their clients, and their communities, and they give of their time to create a positive future for us all. And yet, somehow, they find themselves unable to care for themselves in the ways that *they* need. Now, as I've said repeatedly, I do believe that each of us is responsible for our own thriving, and that we are the best guides on our own health journey. Much of this book has been devoted to showing you how to give that care to yourself. Now, however, it's time to acknowledge that you also need that care from the other people in your life. We *all* do. None of us can walk this path alone.

I used to be convinced that I was strong enough to do it on my own, to continue to show up for others and my responsibilities without help. I even had a kind of martyr complex. It has been such a humbling journey to learn how deluded I really was! It took a lot to open up to and invite support and connection into my healing journey. But now I know that no ingredient is more vital than this.

I now have no doubt that *being held* through this key—Inviting Support and Connection—is one of the most essential, vital elements to creating the life you are here to live, to blossoming and thriving fully as *you*. And yet, sadly, it can be quite elusive for many of us. This key is like the warm embrace that holds the rest of the keys together. Without it, the foundation is shaky. We need each other.

How is it that our health journeys have become so isolated? As we've seen, for so many of us, our relationship with health and self-care is fraught with shame and embarrassment. We often feel all alone in our health struggles—whether it be battling food cravings, trying to lose weight, failing to exercise like we think we ought to, or struggling with a chronic illness day in and day out. We might go to see a doctor occasionally, or we might have some other health practitioners we turn to. But a lot of the time, we're trying to do the best that we can on our own. We compartmentalize our health into a separate box from the rest of our lives. We may actually have a lot of interaction with communities and friends in our lives, but often what's happening for us in regard to health is not shared with the same kind of intimacy as other topics.

One of my clients, Rebecca, a young woman from Chicago, described this sense of isolation poignantly: "I felt like there were nice people around me but I couldn't really connect with them deeply. It was as if we were all moving through life with masks on."

From behind our masks, we might share parts of our story, but not the whole story, not the deeper dimensions where the vulnerability and shame live. In keeping parts of our lives isolated (as our dominant culture encourages us to do), we compound the sense of shame. We feed those voices that say, "Something is wrong with me," or, "Others don't understand or couldn't know what this feels like." We don't realize that everyone else is feeling and thinking the same thing.

Can you imagine how healing it would be if all of this secrecy and isolation were to drop away and we each got to really experience that while our stories and the details of our challenges may be different, there is in fact so much we have in common? We're not all freaks, or as damaged as we might tell ourselves. I have the unique advantage and honor of hearing lots of stories and intimate details of the challenges and struggles people have, and so I know how utterly human we all are. I also know how much we need each other in order to be freed from the struggles we create for ourselves in our isolation. We can't do it alone. Human beings are relational creatures. We need each other.

In her work with me and then in a health mentoring group that I facilitated, Rebecca said that opening up to others felt "magical and kind of unreal." She explained, "I'd never had that experience before. I felt like I had found a place where it was okay to be seen and to be vulnerable."

What made Rebecca ready to take this step after years of hiding behind her mask was the experience of working with the keys outlined in this book, particularly the first key, Honoring Your Unique Life, where she started to come home to herself and her value. When you are truly honoring your unique life your resistance to asking others for help and support will diminish—because of a fierce and newfound loyalty to yourself, you'll do whatever it takes. You're willing to face and embrace the shadows that may have gotten in the way of you reaching out for help in the past. So you can see how the other keys open the door wide for you to invite support and connection into your health journey in a new, life-giving way. And conversely, this key is vital for opening the door wide to all the other keys.

SIX WAYS WE THRIVE THROUGH CONNECTION

In my work I have come to identify six ways in which we thrive in relational support.

1. **REFLECTIONS**: In order to see what we have not been able to see ourselves, we need the perspectives of others. We simply can't see everything about ourselves, by ourselves. There are aspects of ourselves that we are unconscious of. Through relating, we can shine light on what we have not been able to see on our own—an operating system, belief, or paradigm that

we had no idea was running the show. This is why seeking support from others is critical to Key #2, Facing and Embracing Your Shadows.

2. SKILL & CAPACITY BUILDING: If we want to learn the skills and capacities to self-regulate in various ways, we need to seek out the expertise of those who can teach us. From diet, to breath retraining, to somatic practices, to strength training, we can learn so much about how to better care for our bodies and how to increase our self-awareness and knowledge from others who specialize in these areas. This is essential for the third key, Strengthening Your Self-Awareness Muscles, and the fourth key, Cultivating Resilience.

3. GUIDANCE: We don't know what we don't know. We can't see what we have never seen. Others can guide us into new territory, territory *they* have journeyed in but we never knew existed. They can help us to see landmarks, pathways, things to watch out for, things that we may delight in, things that may be of support. Although we each ultimately need to find our way on our own, we also need mentors of some kind to start us on new paths.

4. ACCOUNTABILITY: As I mentioned in the last chapter, if we wish to find our way into discovering easeful discipline so that we can create sustained transformation, we need relational support—there is no ingredient more powerful or essential. A recent weight-loss study by the University of Illinois cited "being accountable to others" as the critical factor in participants' success.[78] And a Stanford University study found that encouraging phone calls with a health educator every three weeks resulted in a 78% increase in exercise for participants compared to a 28% increase for the control group.[79] Changes you struggle to maintain become so much easier when you ask a friend or a practitioner to be an accountability partner. For example, some of my clients will send me text messages or email updates in-between our appointments. It's like magic, the difference it makes. I'll be sharing more suggestions later in this chapter when we talk about peer support.

5. LOVE: Love is really the foundation of this journey. We cannot underestimate the transformative power of love. It allows you to come out of the shame, it saves you from the quicksand of resistance and overwhelm. You are held and nurtured in your movement forward. You are not just out there floundering on your own anymore, or fighting the inner battles that plague so many of us on our health journeys.

And I'm happy to say that medical research is starting to focus more on this very thing! Stanford University's Center for Compassion and Altruism Research and Education (CCARE) teamed up with Dignity Health, a nonprofit public-benefit corporation, to look into the healing power of kindness. Their scientific-literature review states the following:

When patients are treated with kindness—when there is an effort made to get to know them, empathize with them, communicate with them, listen to them and respond to their needs—it can lead to the following outcomes:

✧ faster healing of wounds,

✧ reduced pain,

✧ reduced anxiety,

✧ reduced blood pressure,

✧ and shorter hospital stays.[80]

And of course all of these health benefits can occur outside of a medical context as well! The healing power of kindness, love, and compassion cannot be emphasized enough. In his song "Swim," songwriter Stuart Davis aptly sings, "The only reason that it's scary getting old, / is people treat you like you're too big to hold / and you still feel just like a kid."[81]

Those words pierce my heart every time I hear them. They give voice to the tenderness of our adult journeys, and how we all just yearn, deep down, to be held in unconditional love. While we have our inner Mama Bear to hold ourselves, it isn't the same as when someone else wraps us up in their arms, or gives us their full, undivided loving presence. To be fully heard, honored, and understood by another is such a blessing, and is often at the heart of what wants to be healed.

When I invite my clients to honor the little kid inside them that wants to be held, I watch as time and again something cracks open within them and another defense falls away. They describe a feeling of allowing themselves to really be "seen" and to see themselves. What seems so hard and insurmountable on our own can suddenly seem achievable when held with someone else or a group of people. Sometimes it seems like no big deal at all.

Don't underestimate the power of what love can do. As the great Nelson Mandela writes, "Our human compassion binds us the one to the other—not in pity or patronizingly, but as human beings who have learnt to turn our common suffering into hope for the future."[82]

Sometimes I honestly feel that this loving presence is the heart of what I offer to people through my work. Of course, I have all sorts of knowledge and expertise from my doctoral studies and the lived experience and wisdom born from my own intense healing journey to share, yet when I see the shifts that happen for people in our sessions, they seem to be possible because of the compassion and reliable, steady, loving presence that I offer.

6. PERSPECTIVE: Others remind us that we are not alone. We remember consciously that we are part of the human family, part of a greater whole. Through connection with others, we are reminded that our health journeys are not just about us—they are an integral part of a much bigger picture, of life's unfolding. We'll be returning to this critical perspective in Key #9.

CHECKING IN: *Take a moment to check in with yourself now. As you focus your awareness into this present moment, what is arising? How is this topic of inviting support affecting you in your body, heart, and mind?*

WHO IS ON YOUR SUPPORT TEAM?

The idea of having a *team* of support is key. No one person can provide all the different forms of support that we each need to thrive. Expecting that to be the case only puts unrealistic pressure on that person and sets you up for disappointment and failure.

I've seen repeatedly among my clients how powerful it can be to consciously create a team. Even if you may already have various kinds of support in your life, by consciously identifying the key people and communities who are on your team of support (and making it explicit in your relationships), so much can emerge—greater relaxation and ease, a heightened sense of confidence and empowerment, courage to be vulnerable and real in your process, and a grounded sense that you can indeed achieve what you set out to do.

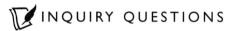

INQUIRY QUESTIONS

Ask yourself these questions as a starting point. Below, I've included several categories that you might want to consider as you design your ideal team of support.

+ What roles would you want on your team? Be specific in describing the parts they each play in the various types of support you need (e.g. professional expertise, forms of accountability, encouragement, guidance, etc.).

+ What qualities, ways of being, skills, or expertise would the people in these roles embody and possess?

+ Who do you already know who might fit these roles?

+ Which roles/people might you need help finding? Who might you ask for recommendations or referrals to find the right people for your team?

+ Who can you reach out to today to begin to build this team?

PEER SUPPORT: This may be one of the easiest and most impactful things that you can start creating, right away. Can you think of a friend who might be in a similar place to you in terms of being ready to create real change, to disentangle from the self-care patterns that haven't been serving him or her so that he or she can blossom and thrive? Invite them to be your "vitality buddy" (or come up with a name that excites you!). It won't cost you anything, and it will not only bring benefit to you, but to your friend, too! In fact, you might have more than one vitality buddy. One you may connect with for exercise, another for emotional support, another for work or life-goal intentions, another for diet, and so on.

Here are some examples of how I have seen clients benefit greatly from peer support. Jack, a client who had great resistance to exercising, found that when he invited his friend (who felt the same way!) to join him, he came to enjoy the movement and received so many benefits that went far beyond the boost in vitality from the exercise itself. The two of them would meet to go for hour-long walks a couple of times a week at a local lake. They began to go biking together. The social time was fun for them both, and their friendship deepened. It also got Jack outside in nature on a regular basis; although this had always been something that nourished him deeply, he'd had trouble motivating himself to get out on his own. With the peer support, the resistance to exercise was no longer an issue.

Another client, Victoria, experimented with using texting as a fun way to connect with her vitality buddy. Every morning they would text their intentions to one another about how they would nourish themselves that day. Then in the evening they would text again to share how it went. It wasn't just about the actions themselves, but about what they learned in the process and how that would inform their next set of intentions and experiments. Then they'd walk together once every week, or every other, and check in at greater length about how they both were doing.

As you can see, the possibilities are endless. You can help each other create new experiments individually and in the form of how you support one another. And you can simply encourage each other. As the Irish poet and philosopher John O'Donohue writes, "One of the most beautiful gifts in the world is the gift of encouragement. When someone encourages you, that person helps you over a threshold you might otherwise never have crossed on your own."[83]

There are, however, a couple of things to watch out for in this kind of support. First, it is very important that this is a *mutually* supportive relationship. If it starts to feel like one person is leaning in more than the other, it may be time to check in and see if perhaps the way in which you are engaging needs to change, or if another type of support needs to come on board. You both will need to be completely honest with each other in this way so that you can relax.

On that note, it is vital that this relationship has proper boundaries. Remember, it is peer support, not professional support. For your own well-being, as well as that of your vitality buddy, be mindful not to overstep your level of expertise, or to expect more from your partner than is realistic. Don't hesitate to suggest professional help if it feels like your partner may need a type of support you cannot offer or that feels uncomfortable for you in any way. Likewise, take responsibility for seeking out the support you need in order to fully enjoy, and benefit from, your peer support.

PARTNER/FAMILY: Just as with peer support, your romantic partner or members of your family can be wonderful partners on your journey toward vitality. Every relationship is unique, however, so I would caution you to have a lot of discernment about what works for you, and what works for your partner and family. Do not assume anything, but instead discover together what is the right level and kind of support that will serve you both.

There are unique advantages to consciously and explicitly adding this kind of support into your romantic relationship. Ideally (and hopefully) you are already cultivating an intimacy in life that includes wanting each other to thrive. Reading a book like this together and sharing your commitments and experiments as you go can be incredibly empowering to you both. If you share a household, it can only add potency to how you can support each other in your processes. Is it by going to the gym together? Shopping for and cooking nourishing meals together? Or planning adventures and vacations that bring you alive? Similarly, if you have kids, you might support each other by sharing in fun play-date adventures with them, learning a new sport as a family, or taking a cooking class all together.

There are also challenges with this kind of support. Since your lives are already so interwoven, it can feel like there is nowhere to just be "you" in your life, to connect with your own process. If your commitments and experiments are explicit in the relationship and you are actively supporting one another, then some shadowy stuff may rise to the surface—the shame, the vulnerability, the self-judgments. This can and will add layers and depth to the intimacy you are already cultivating, and it can, at times, and in some situations, feel like too much too fast, and can destabilize the relationship. Each relationship dynamic is different, so the discernment will have to be up to you. But just as with the peer support, I caution you to clarify your intentions within yourself and between you and your partner. Be mindful to not expect a professional level of support from each other. Ensure that you each have your own *team* on board so that you can love, support, and nourish each other in the ways appropriate for your relationship without putting too much pressure or expectation on a single person.

Remember, also, that no two people are going to be in exactly the same rhythm and readiness in terms of life change and transformation. Just because you are jazzed about what you are reading here and excited about inviting your partner to join you, doesn't mean that they are going to be jazzed, too. You can't force someone to be ready the way that you are, to have the desire to do the things that you want to do. They may be following a different path. You can only take responsibility for yourself and seek out the support you need, and it may not be coming from your partner or family right now. Or perhaps the support you get from them may be simply in loving you no matter how you are or what you are doing.

HEALTHCARE PRACTITIONERS: This is a large category with so many possibilities, especially in today's world, where we're blessed with access to a whole spectrum of healing modalities. Your preferences and your needs will change over time, but having professionals on your team of support is always critical. They not only offer you the expertise of often many years of training, but they also bring the experience of practicing their healing art every day, with a diversity of different people. Thus, they will have skills, perspectives, and a depth of experience that your peer, partner, or family support simply can't offer.

Not only that, but when you go to a health practitioner you are hiring them to be of support to you. This is a one-way relationship in which you can count on them to support you without any other complexities of relationship dynamics getting in the way and without the feeling that you need to reciprocate. They are there for you. They can offer you their expertise, help you learn skills and strengthen your self-awareness, and point you to resources that you can trust. They can help you to hold to your intentions, reflect your values and commitments back to you, support you in revealing your shadows, help you to navigate any stumbles with compassion and grace, guide you in creating new experiments, and remind you that you are in a process that is bigger than yourself.

On my own healing journey, my health-practitioner team of support varied depending on how acute my symptoms were, what I was focused on learning and experimenting with, where I was, and what my resources were. What I came to learn the hard way is that no matter how much training and experience I have as a health practitioner myself, I, too, am a human being

in need of my own team of support. I say that explicitly for all of you reading this who are health practitioners or who have a role in the world that is
in service to caring for others. We *all* need a team of support. We need to
open to being held, to allowing others to be there for us, and allowing their
perspectives to inform us.

At times, I've seen my naturopathic physician every week or two, then
gradually tapered to once a month, then following up as needed. I did the
same thing with an acupuncturist during more acute times of my healing
journey. Because of my training as a massage practitioner and craniosacral
therapist, I've done lots of bodywork trades with other practitioners on a
regular basis, as well as seen a somatic psychotherapist and chiropractor as
needed. I've consulted with many conventional medical doctors and will be
happy to do so again should I need a specialist, or should an emergency medical situation or significant illness arise. I feel open to continuing to listen for
what roles, expertise, and kind of support I may need at any given time and
to find the person or people who seem like a good fit for the respective role.

I know it can be confusing to determine who to invite onto your
health-practitioner team of support, particularly if stepping outside of
mainstream conventional care is new for you. What I've found to be helpful
(and this is a role that I've actually come to embody myself in how I serve
my clients) is to find a health practitioner who can hold the whole picture
with you, who can help you to discern what kinds of support would best
serve you, and who can offer you some referrals as a place to start. That way
you won't be shooting in the dark without the expertise to guide you. In
time, as you try out different practitioners, modalities, and approaches, you
will become more of your own authority in discerning who and what best
supports you at any given time.

It's not always easy to find that person who is willing and able to hold the
big picture of your health and offer compassion and guidance. It might be a
naturopathic physician; it might be some kind of coach, therapist, or medical
advocate; it might be your conventional doctor. You'll have to pay attention
to the different practitioners you encounter, and see who feels like the best fit.
Even though it might be difficult, don't compromise too quickly for a lesser
standard of care. It's a wonderful exercise to let yourself imagine your ideal
health practitioner—to envision his or her qualities without any cynicism
or fear, and to let this vision guide you as you seek members of your team.

The following are some qualities that I look for in the health practi-

tioners I work with (and have focused on cultivating in myself); I offer these
reflections to you here as a way to help you in reflecting on whom you invite
onto your team of support.

I want a health practitioner who . . .

+ Has a loving presence and with whom I feel fully seen and heard—it
feels healing for me simply being around her.

+ Relates with me as one human being to another, owns his humanity,
and doesn't separate himself from me and my experience.

+ Consciously walks her own humble healing journey, so that I can relax
in trusting her to be a guide and mentor for mine.

+ Fully trusts in my capacity to walk my path, and who knows that it is
not his role to direct me, but to offer me the love, support, knowledge,
and expertise that may empower me in my choices on my journey.

Perhaps you have had the opportunity, discernment, and blessing to have
already encountered health practitioners with some or all of these qualities.
Congratulations if that is true for you! If not, I invite you to imagine how
the quality of your healing experience would be affected by inviting health
practitioners onto your team who embody these capacities.

What else would you add to this list for yourself? What qualities, attri-
butes, and skills are most important for your health practitioners to possess?

I'd encourage you to interview health practitioners whom you are considering. Ask them discerning questions and observe not only what they
say, but how they respond and relate to you. Trust your intuition and sense
of resonance or lack thereof. This is an intimate relationship. Just as you
wouldn't invite a lover to your bed whom you didn't resonate with, so, too,
you don't want to invite a health practitioner onto your team of support
whom you do not feel safe and comfortable with.

Remember, Your Doctor Works for You!
While I can't speak to what it is like in other parts of the world, I can quite
confidently say that in the United States, our healthcare system is calling
out for deep healing.

Doctors and health practitioners of all kinds are struggling with burn-out and are caught in a system that doesn't support their own health and well-being or allow them to provide the kinds of care that they know they can (and want to!). When we seek out support on our health journey, it's easy to get caught in the midst of these challenges. We are likely to spend just minutes with our conventional doctors these days, and with the rush it's common to not feel heard, honored, seen, or understood. It can feel like a human being, in this context, gets boiled down to "a forty-two-year-old female with a primary diagnosis of X, Y, or Z." No matter how well-meaning these doctors may be (and most are!), the system they are embedded in makes it extremely difficult for them to get to know who you are as a whole person and appreciate the complexity of what is contributing to your current symptoms and concerns. Therefore, more often than not, a diagnosis just gets a standard protocol of pills, a treatment, further testing, or a referral to a specialist.

It is so very easy to feel intimidated and lack confidence in the face of all of this. Add these things to our cultural tendency to put doctors on a pedestal, and we have a recipe for disempowerment. I've seen this all too often when I've been in the hospital with loved ones—bright, capable people—who were ill. The doctors come in with the few minutes they've been allotted in their busy schedule and try their best to explain what's happening. My loved ones nod along as if they understand it all, then the doctors rush out of the room to their next patient, and they confess they did not understand a word. But did they ask any questions, or ask the doctors to slow down and explain in layman's language? No, they didn't.

Here's what we all need to remember, no matter who we are, what our training is, or who we are consulting with: YOU are in charge of your health journey. When you go to a healthcare professional, you are hiring them to support you. They are your consultant—you are paying them to do a treatment or therapy for you. This is true regardless of whether insurance is involved or not. This can help you to stay autonomous and not forget that you are actually your own best health guide. Nobody else but you is living with you 24/7 and receiving all of the feedback and symptoms. Only you can discern what brings you alive and what doesn't. As you develop these self-care capacities, you will have more confidence with your healthcare practitioners. You will more easily be able to ask them their opinions and receive treatments without letting go of your power, because you recognize that you are in charge. Be the boss. Seek out the answers you need. Make sure that no one deflects your questions—if they do they are probably not the best person to have on your team of support.

You have many options for choosing health practitioners who will support and honor you and your needs. We each are unique and will resonate with different approaches, personalities, and settings.

MEDICAL ADVOCATES: Although, as I've repeatedly said in this book, you are your own best health guide, there will be times when you are simply not able to fulfill this role. If you are suffering a serious illness, you may not always be in a position to take in and rationally weigh up your choices and options. At moments like this, you may need someone else to act as a medical advocate for you—to ask the questions, keep track of your journey, and help you to navigate when you are in the throes of pain and fear. This person could be a friend or a loved one, or a professional advocate you can turn to in times of need.

COMMUNITY OF PRACTICE: I have come to be a huge proponent of "communities of practice," a term that was coined by anthropologists Jean Lave and Etienne Wenger in the 1980s to refer to communities that engage in processes of collective learning, or "groups of people who share a concern or a passion for something they do and learn how to do it better as they interact regularly."[84]

Sadly, these are not all that common in healthcare outside of addiction support groups, so most people have not benefited from all that they offer. In the context of embodying and integrating the nine keys in this book into your daily life, you can accelerate and deepen your learning and healing by being part of a community of practice. Here are some ways you might seek out communities of practice:

+ Think about your close friends: are there three or four people you might invite to join you in a group?

+ Ask your health practitioners if they know of local groups.

+ If you're a member of a church or spiritual community, see if there are support groups connected to it.

✦ If you're looking for support for specific issues, like weight loss or addiction, you can search online for local support groups.

Here are a couple of recommendations to guide you in creating or finding a community of practice (see the Appendix for more guidance):

✦ If you are creating your own community of practice, it is important to get very clear about your intentions and to make sure those intentions are clear among everyone participating. Different groups can have very different types of focus.

✦ If you are inviting friends to join you in creating a group, it is important that you differentiate your community-of-practice times of engagement from times when you are just getting together socially. Create a regular structure that is clear and that you can all commit to.

✦ Depending on what kind of community of practice you have created, you may want to consider hiring an outside facilitator to support your process. Alternatively, you can choose one member of your group to facilitate, or rotate the facilitators each time you meet in a way that empowers everyone in the group to step into leadership.

✦ If you are seeking out a community of practice in your local community or online, I'd encourage you to treat it the same as if you were interviewing health practitioners. There are so many different kinds of groups, facilitators, and approaches. Don't be shy about trying groups out and moving on if it is not the right fit. Trust that you will know when it feels deeply resonant and safe for you to be held in that particular community container.

In their book *Wellbeing*, Tom Rath and Jim Harter present research that validates the importance of working in this kind of community:

Experimental research suggests that creating sustainable change may be two to three times as likely to happen in the context of a group, company, or community organization. For example, if you enroll in an intensive weight-loss program alone, there is a 24% chance that you will maintain your weight loss after 10 months. If you enroll in the same program and then join a social support group of three strangers, there is a nearly 50% chance you will maintain the weight loss 10 months later. But if you enroll in the program with three friends or colleagues you already know, the odds of maintaining your weight loss go up to 66%.[85]

I first came to realize the healing power of this kind of community experience when I was a participant in groups that were not framed around healing. They were about developing leadership skills or spiritual growth. Yet, because I participated in these programs in the midst of my healing journey, I saw what happened as a result of being in them. I saw my energy increase, my nervous system relax, my inspiration in life expand, my clarity of purpose ignite, and I felt myself become more comfortable and at home in who I was and who I was becoming. I felt more alive and at ease in life. And as I observed the other participants I saw similar patterns, even if there was often a bumpy transitional period in the transformation and growth that was happening.

There's something almost magical that happens when we are held in a collective where it is safe to be vulnerable, to face and embrace our shadows, to let ourselves be seen in the raw, humble beauty of our imperfect humanness. Rebecca, the client who I mentioned earlier in the chapter, described her experience of community as "an antidote to everything my depressed mind was saying about me." After working with the group for the first time, she realized, "Everybody suffers. It made the whole difficult situation I was in feel like a gift, because it revealed my interconnectedness with all of humanity. It was such a relief to have others hold me for a change. I am used to shouldering everything on my own."

The benefits that I had had from previous community-practice experiences led me to join a somatic-therapy group in 2009, which proved to be an enormous source of support and insight as I engaged with my own shadows. This group, led by an incredibly embodied, skillful, and gifted practitioner, has been, for me, an amazing gift of continuity, offering me the same intimate group to work with for all this time. We meet every three months for a weekend intensive, and it is deep! This group has supported me in revealing and healing the underbelly of my fatigue and coming home to who I am here to be.

Through this work I've come to embrace and own anger, fear, and other emotions that were not modeled for me in a healthy way when I was growing up. I've explored the insecurities, shame, judgments, and coping patterns I have had around my sexuality and romantic relationships. I've touched into such young, tender, terrified parts of myself. I've revealed to this loving cohort parts of myself that I didn't even know were there, parts that were so very vulnerable to feel, let alone reveal to others. And what is incredible is that not only was I doing this kind of work, but the ten other members of my group were also revealing themselves in these same raw and tender ways. I can't tell you how grateful I am to have had this opportunity to be completely and unapologetically human with a group of people. I'm reminded of poet Adrienne Rich's words: "No person, trying to take responsibility for her or his identity, should have to be so alone. There must be those among whom we can sit down and weep, and still be counted as warriors."[86]

When I talk about a community of practice around your healing, I'm not just talking about any kind of community. There are particular qualities and commitments that need to be a part of such a community so that it is safe, honoring, and truly supportive. You need to be discerning that the person or people leading the group have done enough of their own healing work (as participants) to have the capacity to be with people in their raw vulnerability and shame; in the tender, young parts; in the woundedness; and in the golden shadows that are waiting to be revealed. You need to trust that they know how to guide you and the whole group toward the vitality and healing that is in the center of all of that.

In addition, the participants in the group need to be in a place in themselves where they can hold the process with confidentiality and deep honor for having the opportunity to support and witness others in their vulnerability. The vulnerability is woven into every aspect of healing, and part of what keeps us stuck in our capacity to create the change we seek is in not acknowledging the deeper levels of what is calling out for healing. Rarely does a surface-level habit change result in sustained change without the deeper work.

I am continually amazed how much we can open and shine, and how freely we can move forward, when we witness others, are witnessed by others, and share ourselves in community. The reason that so many of my programs are designed for intimate groups whose members can support one another over time is for this very reason. There is nothing else like it when it comes to sustaining change in our lives.

So much of what keeps us stuck on our health journeys can be freed up in being in an intimate community that is held with consciousness and guided by intentionality. Why? Because we can finally see that we are not alone. Others can totally understand what we are going through (even if they haven't experienced exactly the same thing). Yes, we all are living unique lives, but shared human themes and patterns underlie the details of our experiences. In community we are able to reveal and see the deeper layers and witness and love each other into our healing.

STAYING CONNECTED TO YOUR OWN AUTHORITY, STRENGTH AND INNER WISDOM

Turning to others for support is not about handing over authority. I think a lot of us fear reaching out for support because we equate it with being weak or giving over our power. In my experience it is the opposite. When we find those whom we trust to bring onto our team of support, we access a new strength—one that we can find only in the vulnerability of being transparent, being seen in our wholeness, revealing the parts of ourselves that we may be ashamed of or embarrassed about.

And as you may remember from Keys #3 and #4, when we take the time to cultivate an intimacy with and mastery of our own body-homes, we feel clear and strong in ourselves. This allows us to show up in relationship with others from a place of security and confidence. And when we are in charge of ourselves in this way, we can filter others' reflections, knowledge, and expertise—we can feel what resonates and what doesn't. We can take in what supports us and let the rest go.

Recognizing that you need support and then asking for that is a huge and empowering step. There comes a point on any path of personal development where you recognize that you simply cannot afford *not* to invest in your own transformation and healing. What that looks like is very different for each of us. But every one of us matters and is worth the investment. Investment isn't all about money. It's also about where we focus our time and energy, what we prioritize, and who we invite into our lives.

In this spirit of valuing and honoring yourself, I wanted to emphasize again how important it is to have discernment and self-respect about whom you share your vulnerabilities with and whom you invite onto your team of support. As Brené Brown cautions, "If we share our shame story with the wrong person, they can easily become one more piece of flying debris in an already dangerous storm."[87] However, she also writes, "If we can share our story with someone who responds with empathy and understanding, shame can't survive."[88] Choose people to be on your team who have the capacity to hold all of who you are—your darkness and your light—and to embrace the complexity, nuance, and ups and downs of the journey *with* you, while practicing love, gentleness, and compassion. They are not there to fix you, but to be of support to you. They understand that *you* are in charge of your own journey. However, they also understand that sharing the journey with you will make the road easier for you *and* for them, while moving you both toward greater health and vitality.

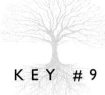

KEY #9

LIVING LIKE
YOU MATTER

"Don't ask yourself what the world needs.
Ask yourself what makes you come alive and then go do that.
Because what the world needs is people who have come alive."
—HOWARD THURMAN

"IF YOU HAD told me, back when I first sat down with you, that someday I would be grateful for what I went through, I would have thought you were crazy!" Kathy laughed out loud. Her joy, vitality, and gratitude were contagious and I found myself laughing too, while my mind scanned back to that day when we first met, a little over a year before. I could hardly believe how far she had come.

The woman who had entered my office that day the previous year had been barely hanging on to her sanity and health. She was fifty-one, but looked years older. She told me she had recently made the shocking discovery that her husband whom she had been with for thirty-five years had been having an affair. Initially unable to let herself feel how angry she was at him, she'd turned her anger on herself, for not having seen what was going on in front of her eyes. Desperately trying to keep it together for her teenage kids, she felt hopelessly ill-equipped to navigate life on her own. Added to all this was her father's cancer diagnosis. "I'm in so much pain," she'd told me then, "that I'm not able to give to my kids and my dad in the way that I want to, and at the same time I feel like I'm giving them more than I am able to give."

What struck me most about Kathy's story was her description of how she felt when she contemplated moving forward in life without her husband. "I feel as though without him in my life that part of my life would disappear, the thirty-five years would just be gone. There are little moments of awareness that my life can still have a lot of meaning and I will be okay, but I can't fully fathom that, because being with him is all I have ever known. I have been with him since I was sixteen."

For Kathy to learn to care for herself, she first had to learn to be herself, independent from her marriage. After creating as much space as she needed for her grief, I helped her to clarify what she wanted in all the different areas of her life. "It feels really scary to even think about creating my own life, about what I want to be" she told me. "I've only ever asked, 'What do all the people around me need me to be?'"

Kathy explored the terrain of all of the first eight keys, including learning to value herself, to acknowledge her own repressed anger, to listen to her body and respond and experiment, and to find structures of support and community. Slowly, she began to learn "to be in touch with myself, with my own emotion and truth, rather than always turning to other people. I learned to tune into my own voice. I came to see that how I feel is valid." Kathy recognized that through the years of her marriage, there had been a "slow process of wearing down my self-esteem and losing who I was. And I allowed that to happen. Through our work together, I needed to unravel it and start working towards an authentic life."

Today, the woman who sits with me looks even younger than her fifty-two years. She's powerful, grounded, full of energy, and deeply attuned with herself and her own nourishment. She tells me that she's been attending community college and has now applied for her BA—something she had put off in order to support her husband in his education and then raise their children.

"What are you planning to study?" I ask.

"Counseling," she replies. "I want to work with women who are in times of transition. Every time I tune into that now, it simply feels good in my body. It feels right. I know what it is that I'm here to do and that's the direction I'm going. I feel that clearly, even when other people have questioned my decision. I don't know all the specifics, all I know is that if I put my intelligence out there to the universe, and I walk towards that, it will fall into place. And that brings joy and peace and a sense of connection to the sacred and a sense of purpose.

"It also tells me that all my life experiences have got me here to what I am doing. I wouldn't be on this path if I had not gone through the experience that I went through. So as strange as it sounds even to me as I say it, I am truly grateful for the experience that happened. I never, ever thought that I would feel that way."

The alignment that had occurred in Kathy's life was tangible. This woman, who had had a classic case of the Bodhisattva Syndrome—giving everything to others and losing herself—had now found herself, and found a way to serve and give back that did not conflict with her self-care, but, in fact, nourished her more and more deeply. Kathy had naturally become an expression of Key #9: Living Like You Matter.

Just as they did for Kathy, the other eight keys have paved the way to lead you here, to the ninth key, Living Like You Matter. This path I've been guiding you on, in fact this entire book, is an invitation, a call to action for you to consciously cultivate the foundation in yourself that you need to serve the world. Put simply, *your health isn't just about you.*

We are living in a time of such rapid change with so much complexity and challenges that we have never encountered before. We face stark realities as a human family that we simply cannot ignore. I believe that whether we are conscious of it or not, each and every one of us, in every moment, is playing our part in life's unfolding. And life has never needed each one of us, in all our uniqueness and vitality, as much as it does today.

With the tools I've been sharing in this book, I hope I can support you in being able to answer that call in a way that is deeply aligned and congruent with your own thriving—a way that is not only personally sustainable but even contributes to your flourishing. Each and every one of us is a vital player in creating a positive future for us all; we each have a role to play. And in order to support our collective and planetary well-being, each of us needs to be as strong, clear, and vital as we can be.

Living Like You Matter is about finally healing the split between self-care and our service and contribution in the world. It's the answer to the Bodhisattva Syndrome; or, put another way, it's the way to become a true Bodhisattva. We can become, with the help of this key, the Bodhisattvas who do not forsake ourselves. We include our own welfare in our service. We choose to live our lives in compassionate service to life itself.

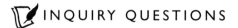 INQUIRY QUESTIONS

Let's pause for a moment now so you can have a chance to reflect on what all of this means for you. Grab your journal and take whatever time you need to contemplate the following questions:

+ What does healing the split between self-care and your service in the world look like for you?

+ Where do you tend to sacrifice yourself in order to serve others or a greater cause? Is it in your family? With your partner? With friends? In your work? In communities you engage with? In your personal and professional development?

+ In what ways do you prioritize the needs of others above your own?

+ What are the current impacts on your daily life of these behaviors?

+ What do you see as the longer-term impacts if you continue with these patterns?

+ What might your life look like if you no longer sacrificed yourself in order to serve?

Life needs you to be here flourishing as you. We all need you to invest in cultivating an intimate and empowered foundation to how you live, relate, breathe, and serve. *No one else on this planet but you can make that happen.* And we are all relying on you to do that, for each of us to do that, for ourselves.

If you're feeling unsure whether this really applies to you, please consider what psychologist and wilderness guide Bill Plotkin beautifully says: "Remember that self-doubt is as self-centered as self-inflation. Your obligation is to reach as deeply as you can and offer your unique and authentic gifts as bravely and beautifully as you're able."[89] True service is rooted in nourishing your body and your being, stewarding yourself toward the most alive, vital version of you, so that you can unleash your unique creative offering on the world. And it all feeds back—you will come more alive in offering your unique gifts, in aligning more closely with your "yes!" and supporting your unique expression to flourish.

A WEB OF VITALITY

"To regain our full humanity," writes physicist Fritjof Capra, "we have to regain our experience of connectedness with the entire web of life."[90] We are all unique expressions of life that are parts of the greater whole. When we begin to live from truly knowing that as a universal truth, not just intellectually but through a felt connection, the distinctions between personal, collective, and planetary health drop away. In his book *The Web of Life*, Capra describes "a holistic worldview, seeing the world as an integrated whole rather than a dissociated collection of parts . . . not as a collection of isolated objects, but as a network of phenomena that are fundamentally interconnected and interdependent."[91] What we might call a part, he explains, "is merely a pattern in an inseparable web of relationships."[92]

As you engage with Key #9, you will come to see through your lived experience how every element of this universe interpenetrates and informs every other element. Your own vitality is impacted by the vitality around you in other people, nature, and the world. And the vitality around you is influenced by the vitality within you, by your state of aliveness.

As the vibration of vitality around us increases, so, too, are more of us able to realize the ease of aliveness available to us on a personal level. I'm sure you have experienced this when you have spent time in the wilderness, or have gone to a beautiful park in the middle of a city. You might have felt your body relax, your mind clear, and a dynamic sense of ease come into your whole being as you received the reflection of the vitality of life around you. Or perhaps you have had the joy of witnessing the unfettered exuberance of a young child, and noticing how quickly this can ignite your own vitality and playfulness. Life around you and life within you are in a constant interplay, feeding and nourishing the other in an endless back and forth.

Likewise, I imagine you have felt the impact on your state of being if you've spent time in places that have suffered extreme environmental devastation, or with people who are malnourished, or with a loved one who is severely depressed. We are affected by the life-energies of the people and places around us. And we affect those around us, too!

Have you ever experienced yourself in a really alive state of being coming into contact with those who might be more subdued, ill, or just not as awake in that moment? Something happens, simply by you being in your enlivened state. You begin to see them emerge from whatever state they were in. Their eyes take on more of a glow. They may begin to smile and laugh for the first time in a while. Their cheeks may gain more color. They may start to show curiosity and wonder about things outside of what they had been focused on before. And all that has happened is that you have shown up with presence, with your natural vitality shining through. It is contagious! Why? Because we all have the same life-energy inside of us. Our vibrations reverberate with each other. As American mythologist Joseph Campbell says, "The influence of a vital person vitalizes, there's no doubt about that."[93]

What I've come to see is that as we come more alive in ourselves, when we encounter *dis*-ease around us, it naturally ignites our vital engagement and dynamic contribution. Not in a way that we become depleted but in a way that we come more alive in offering ourselves in service to the whole through sharing our unique gifts, whatever they may be, and at whatever level we are drawn to engage. As the distinguished physician Larry Dossey so eloquently says, "When our focus is toward a principle of relatedness and oneness, and away from fragmentation and isolation, health ensues."[94]

By supporting the healing of others and our planet, we are also healing ourselves, and in healing ourselves, we are supporting the healing of others and our planet. As our awareness expands to recognize our intrinsic place in the greater whole of life, we naturally look inward as much as we look outward because we recognize our own participation as being a vital part of life. The two are intimately intertwined. As Kathy puts it, "I'm much more in tune to what nurtures me and I'm really good at giving myself those things. I really am understanding how vital it is that I do that and that the more I do that the more I become authentic and the more I can be a conduit of joy and gratitude and love for people around me." You, too, can cultivate your skills and capabilities in these ways. You know now from your exploration of the other keys that you have the capacity to expand your self-awareness, to attune to the feedback you are receiving all the time that is letting you know when you are thriving or out of balance and in *dis*-ease. As you cultivate this awareness and weave in the skills of self-regulation, you are able to guide and align yourself with your own felt aliveness and flourishing.

As you begin to engage with this final key, Living Like You Matter, you can discover that you have these same innate capacities when tuning into life around you. You have the opportunity, in encountering *dis*-ease around you—in other people, your community, and the planet at large—to cultivate the awareness and skills to contribute to guiding others and life as a whole toward greater vitality. If you can't access that capacity right away, don't worry. All you have to do, like Kathy did, is to listen to your own needs and continue to respond to what your inner voice yearns for. The beauty of this key is that in fully nurturing yourself, you will free up your own energy and attention to respond naturally to the needs of the world around you. It's not something you need to force. The invitation here is to simply open yourself to this process and, in so doing, become a conscious part of guiding all of life toward vital, vibrant health.

🎧 **WEB OF LIFE MEDITATION:** *I'd like to invite you now to join me on a guided meditation journey. Begin by simply inviting yourself home into your body. See if you can allow yourself to feel all of the different dimensions of your consciousness—your emotions, thoughts, and the physical sensations that arise. Tune into the data and feedback that is there all the time. Let yourself simply scan your body and feel all the different sensations that are letting you know that you are in a body right now—the tensions, places of ease, your breath that is naturally cycling, feeding, and nourishing you. Acknowledge the intricate body systems that keep life pulsing through you. Drop deeper to see if you can feel the subtle pulsation of your heart moving blood through your entire body system. And feel beneath that to see if you can touch into the even subtler pulsations that are there. You might not be able to name it, or even be able to describe it to anyone. Yet even so, see if you can drop into the level of feeling the subtle pulsation of life infusing you. You are alive! Can you contact that in this moment—can you feel how brief, precious, and wondrous it is to be alive and in a body, right now?*

As you stay connected to a felt sense of your own body in this way, I'd like you to think of a few people who are part of your daily life—your family, close friends, your inner circle. Close your eyes and see if you can feel a direct connection with them. Imagine a thread connecting you to them. Allow yourself to feel the love and care and perhaps the complexity of other emotions that are there, too, as you allow your awareness to connect with them.

Now expand your awareness to take in people who are part of your social circles, to one by one feel and see the thread of connection with the people who come into your consciousness. They might live close by, or across the globe, be part of your professional world, or dear friends. Notice whatever may arise for you as you bring these beings into your awareness.

Now expand your awareness even further to take in the greater human family of which you are a part. Consciously reach out to people who you might not have ever met, people who you pass on the street, people who live in a country you may have never visited. And, again, open to allowing yourself to feel and see the threads of connection that are there, however you experience it in this moment, to these other members of the human species, your human family.

Now imagine yourself sitting in a beautiful spot in nature, whatever feels nurturing to you. Perhaps it is a grove of trees, with sun filtering through. Or perhaps it is a tropical beach, or a mountain peak. As you keep the sense of connection with your human family, of being part of a web made up of all those threads of connection, I'd like you to open your senses to take in this natural scene in which you are sitting. Feel how the air is touching your skin, hear the textures of the sounds, the movements of the various life forms, birds, insects, rodents scurrying across the ground, the wind in the trees. Allow your senses to take it all in: the sounds, smells, and tactile experiences. Open your eyes to clearly see this alive, natural scene. Allow yourself to observe the life-force infusing all of life around you—the magic and vibrancy of that. As you observe you are able to take in the natural cycle of things flourishing and coming alive and the impermanence of that. You can see how the plants, animals, birds, and insects are unselfconsciously thriving in their habitats, how utterly natural that is. See if you can sense the threads of connection with the life around you in the same way that you were able to with the human beings you reached out to.

As you connect with the reflections of nature, feeling the connections with the greater human family, return to the pulsation of life-energy inside of you. You are infused with the same life-energy of all you are taking in, all those people, the members of the human family that you were connecting with. And it is the same life-energy infusing all of the animals and plants around you.

CHECKING IN: *As you come out of the meditation, take a deep breath and reconnect with your body in this moment. How are you able to sense the* *life-energy pulsing through you now? Where in your body do you tap into the sense of inner guidance—your heart, your gut, your throat, your solar plexus? What is your guidance telling you right now?*

FILLING YOUR PLACE

We each have a particular role to play in the drama of life. We each need to do our part in serving the greater whole. As physician and author Deepak Chopra so beautifully says, "There are no extra pieces in the universe. Everyone is here because he or she has a place to fill, and every piece must fit itself into the big jigsaw puzzle."[95] Whatever it is that we are each here to experience and bring forward as our gift and contribution is not only worthy and valid: it is absolutely necessary. In simply being alive we embody an innate sense of worth. *We each matter!* We don't have to prove anything.

The impulse to create, to share ourselves, to put something out there in the world to be received, feels akin to a bud bursting open into a glorious flower. No matter who sees that flower, there is an innate celebration of life expressing itself, simply in the process of blossoming. Just like the plants and creatures in the meditation we just experienced, we all have the opportunity to unselfconsciously and naturally thrive. We all have that possibility to flourish, blossom, and come into that fullest expression of ourselves simply because we are here. It is implicitly and explicitly a part of being alive—the most essential, innate invitation of life.

INQUIRY QUESTIONS

What is life inviting you to become? What is your part in the dance of creation? Here are a few more questions to guide your integration of this final key, Living Like You Matter. These are questions that you can return to over and over, as you and all of life continues to evolve:

+ What does "living like you matter" mean to you?

+ What are your biggest concerns for the health and flourishing of our human family? What about for other life and our planet?

◆ What, if anything, do you feel called to in terms of your unique service or contribution toward addressing these challenges? What are you willing to devote your life to?

◆ What gifts might you have to share, and at what scale are you drawn to share them?

◆ What might be an experiment you could try out to explore how your own sense of vitality may be interconnected with the ways in which you show up to serve others?

◆ How might you align your ways of serving others with your own self-care so that you come more fully alive in your creative offering?

◆ What's one action step that you could take today to step more fully into living like you matter?

Don't worry if you can't answer all of these questions right away. What matters is simply that you give yourself the space and the freedom to ask them, and that you begin to take action when the answers naturally reveal themselves. If you are worried that you can't handle anything more on your plate right now, just remember that this key, Living Like You Matter, is not about self-sacrifice. Trust that if you continue to care for yourself and nourish your unique expression, you will find a natural and sustainable way for that light to shine into the world.

Letting that light shine is your greatest responsibility. If you allow your shining to be subdued, or your thread to become weak or to break, the entire web of life feels it. Your vibrations of life-energy and expression move through the web of life all the time. When you are more juicy and alive you send bigger reverberations out into the web. It doesn't matter if your focus is on your family, your local community, or on the larger systems at play in our world. When you come more alive that energy ripples out through the web. Can you feel the potential if you were to truly unleash your force of love and creative goodness in the world?

And please remember that your flourishing, your contribution, your thriving in life may very well include pathology and illness. Living Like You Matter is about wholeheartedly standing in your authenticity, accepting and bringing forth what is uniquely yours to experience and offer. For many of us (myself certainly included!), illness can be an incredible, awakening, life-giving journey that invites us to live in greater alignment with the heart of who we are here to be. Our life transformation and our conscious engagement with what life brings us, whatever it may be, is all part of our flourishing.

MY WISHES FOR YOU, AND FOR ALL OF US

As this book comes to a close, I want to leave you with some heartfelt wishes I have for you. They are the same wishes I have for myself, and for all of us in our human family.

I wish for you to move through life with more vitality, ease, and love—for yourself, for those intimate to you, for those in the human family whom you may never meet, for all of life, and for this planet that holds us.

I wish for you to have the courage to take a strong stand for your life, to commit to cultivating a reality for yourself that allows you to blossom in the world.

I wish for you to feel a sweet joy, awe, and gratitude for the honor of guiding and nourishing yourself into the fullness and depth of the vitality that is your birthright.

I wish for you to share your aliveness with others, letting it ripple out in the presence you offer, in the capacities you share, in the living reminder you become of what really matters in life.

I wish for you to invite playfulness and joy along for the ride in this mysterious, beautiful journey of life.

And I wish for you to give yourself the gift of compassion, nurturing, and healing so that you can give life the gift of more of you!

What do *you wish* for?

APPENDIX

*A Guide to Facilitating Your Own
Vitality Map Community of Practice*

The following are suggestions for how you might create a community of practice to work with the principles in *The Vitality Map*.

1. GATHER YOUR COMMUNITY

✦ Create a clear intention statement about what you would like to create and why that you can use to invite your friends and community to join you.

✦ You might revisit Key #8 to recall the qualities that you are looking for in the people you invite to join so that the community of practice can offer you (and everyone in it) the support that will serve you best. This is a time to have discernment and clarity so that when you share your invitation, you attract people who are ripe and ready in the same ways that you are!

✦ I'd suggest keeping the group to around six people—a large enough group to ensure varied input and perspectives and to allow for the experience of momentum that happens in a group context, yet small enough for everyone to receive personalized attention and support.

✦ You'll need to decide whether you want this to be a local group that meets in person or a virtual community that meets via video calls on a platform like Skype or Google Hangouts.

2. CREATE YOUR SCHEDULE

✦ I'd suggest having ten sessions. Meet at the frequency that works best for you—weekly, every other week, or monthly for 1.5–2 hours at a time, depending on the size of the group.

◆ Each session will focus on a specific chapter or set of chapters of *The Vitality Map*. You can have everyone read the chapter(s) and do the inquiry questions and practical exercises prior to meeting, with the following schedule:

⬥ Session 1: Focus on the content and practical exercises in the Introduction and Chapters 1-3.

⬥ Sessions 2–10: Devote one session to each of the 9 Keys to Deep Vitality, progressing in chronological order through the book.

3. CLARIFY YOUR COMMITMENTS TOGETHER

◆ Set aside 20 to 30 minutes in the first meeting to clarify your commitments both individually and as a community so that the group becomes a strong, clear, safe container in which you can all relax and engage.

◆ Some topics you might discuss:

⬥ Confidentiality agreements;

⬥ What you each want to be held accountable for in the process;

⬥ Whether you want to add anything else to the process, such as another layer of support in the form of vitality buddies, so that group members can check in with each other between community sessions (via text, email, a walk, or phone call);

⬥ How you want to structure your meetings;

⬥ Whether you want to rotate the role of facilitator or if the initiator of the group will maintain the facilitator role.

4. STRUCTURE THE FLOW OF YOUR MEETINGS

✦ For a 2-hour meeting with six participants, you might structure it like this:

 ◇ 10 minutes: Start with a grounding exercise: a silent or guided meditation or some movement to help everyone settle consciously into their bodies.

 ◇ 90 minutes: Take turns sharing, allocating 15 minutes for each person. 10 minutes of that might be uninterrupted sharing—what they've been learning and applying from the chapter and exercises, what they are struggling with, and what they have to celebrate (this is important to include!). Then 5 minutes for feedback, reflections, and shared learning from the group. I'd encourage you to help each other to go deep in order to touch into more vulnerable territory that each chapter will help unveil. This aspect of the community experience is what will support profound growth for all participants.

 ◇ 10 minutes: People can share whatever other learning or insights might have come from witnessing each other's process. (We can learn so much from each other!)

 ◇ 10 minutes: Close the meeting by inviting each person to state clear intentions and/or next steps that they are taking with them from the session. Try to keep these intentions and steps practical and grounded in the realities of daily life and tied to the larger process of *The Vitality Map*.

5. CLARIFY NEXT STEPS

✦ As your 10 sessions come to a close, clarify whether you want to create any kind of ongoing structure to support each person in continuing to deepen into the long-term life practices that *The Vitality Map* has introduced. Take time to brainstorm. Perhaps you will decide to have ongoing vitality buddies, a monthly check in with the whole group, an online forum in which to share with one another (like a private Facebook group)—or maybe at some point you'll want to create another 10-session community journey with *The Vitality Map*.

I want to be of support to you in this process! If you'd like further free resources to assist you in creating or participating in a Vitality Map Community of Practice, go to **www.thevitalitymap.com/communityofpractice** (or scan the QR code below).

ENDNOTES

1. Leslie Kwoh, "When the CEO Burns Out," *The Wall Street Journal*, May 7, 2013, wsj.com.

2. Arianna Huffington, *Thrive* (Harmony, 2014), Kindle edition, 30.

3. Huffington, *Thrive*, 35–36.

4. Ibid., 30.

5. Brené Brown, *Daring Greatly: How the Courage to Be Vulnerable Transforms the Way We Live, Love, Parent, and Lead* (Avery, 2012), Kindle edition, 69.

6. Brown, *Daring Greatly*, 86.

7. Ibid., 33–34.

8. Ibid., 39–40.

9. Michael Finkelstein, *Slow Medicine* (William Morrow, 2015), 10.

10. Adyashanti, *Falling into Grace* (Sounds True, 2011), Kindle edition, 229.

11. Jacqueline Olds, MD, and Richard S. Schwartz, MD, *The Lonely American* (Beacon Press, 2009), 16.

12. "Missing the Healthcare Connection," The American Psychological Association, accessed May 26, 2015, http://www.apa.org/news/press/releases/stress/2012/health-care.aspx.

13. Huffington, *Thrive*, 14.

14. Paulo Coelho, *The Pilgrimage* (Plus) (HarperCollins, 2009), Kindle edition, 40–41.

15. Ibid., 35.

16. Steven Pressfield, *The War of Art* (Black Irish Entertainment LLC, 2011), Kindle edition, 123.

17. Joanna Macy, "Personal Guidelines for the Great Turning," accessed May 26, 2015, http://www.joannamacy.net/personal-guidelines.html.

18. Rachel Naomi Remen, "Healing Yourself," accessed May 26, 2015, http://www.rachelremen.com/learn/self-care.

19. Mary Oliver, "The Summer Day" from *New and Selected Poems* (Beacon Press, 1992).

20. A. Mille, *Martha: The Life and Work of Martha Graham* (Random House, 1991), 264.

21. Bell Hooks, *All About Love* (Harper Perennial, 2000), 68.

22. Bernie S. Siegel, *Love, Medicine and Miracles: Lessons Learned about Self-Healing from a Surgeon's Experience with Exceptional Patients* (HarperCollins, 2011), Kindle edition, 67–68.

23. Bruce Greyson, "Near-death experience: clinical implications," *Archives of Clinical Psychiatry* (São Paulo), 34 (Supl. 1), 116–125 (2007).

24. Gabrielle Roth, *Maps to Ecstasy: A Healing Journey for the Untamed Spirit* (New World Library, 2011), 142.

25. C. G. Jung, *Collected Works of C.G. Jung*, Volume 9 (Part 2): Aion: Researches into the Phenomenology of the Self (Kindle Locations 4693-4695) (Princeton University Press, 2014), Kindle Edition.

26. Steven Pressfield, *The War of Art* (Black Irish Entertainment LLC, 2011), Kindle Edition, 12.

27. C. G. Jung, *Collected Works of C.G. Jung*, Volume 9 (Part 2): Aion: Researches into the Phenomenology of the Self (Kindle Locations 4703-4705) (Princeton University Press, 2014), Kindle Edition.

28. Marianne Williamson, *Everyday Grace* (Riverhead Books, 2002), 12–13.

29. John E. Sarno, *The Divided Mind* (HarperCollins, 2009), Kindle Edition, 12.

30. Maggie Craddock, *The Authentic Career: Following the Path of Self-Discovery to Professional Fulfillment* (New World Library, 2010), 54.

31. Gabor Mate, *When the Body Says No* (Vintage Canada, 2003), 246.

32. Ibid, 247.

33. Rachel Naomi Remen, *Kitchen Table Wisdom* (Penguin Group, 2006), 37–38.

34. Byron Katie, *Loving What Is: Four Questions That Can Change Your Life* (Three Rivers Press, 2003), 3.

35. C. G. Jung, Letters, Volume 2 (Princeton University Press, 1973), 234.

36. Hal Stone, PhD, and Sidra Stone, PhD, "Voice Dialogue: Discovering Our Selves," http://delos-inc.com/articles/Voice_Dialogue_Discovering_Our_Selves.pdf.

37. Ibid.

38. J. Krishnamurti, *Choiceless Awareness 1* (M-Y Books Ltd, 2012).

39. Julia Cameron, *The Artist's Way* (Penguin Publishing Group, 2002), Kindle Edition, 572–73.

40. Mihaly Csikszentmihalyi, *Flow: The Psychology of Optimal Experience* (Harper Perennial, 1991), 24.

41. Brian Walker and David Salt, *Resilience Thinking: Sustaining Ecosystems and People in a Changing World* (Island Press, 2006), 9.

42. David S. Olton and Aaron R. Noonberg, *Biofeedback: Clinical Applications in Behavioral Medicine* (Prentice-Hall, 1980), 4.

43. Volker Busch, MD, Walter Magerl, MD, Uwe Kern, MD, Joachim Haas, MD, Göran Hajak, MD, and Peter Eichhammer, MD. 2012. *The Effect of Deep and Slow Breathing on Pain Perception, Autonomic Activity, and Mood Processing—An Experimental Study.* Pain Medicine. 13: 215–228.

44. Chacko N. Joseph, Cesare Porta, Gaia Casucci, Nadia Casiraghi, Mara Maffeis, Marco Rossi, Luciano Bernardi. 2005. *Slow Breathing Improves Arterial Baroreflex Sensitivity and Decreases Blood Pressure in Essential Hypertension.* Hypertension. 46: 714-718.

45. Gabor Maté, *When the Body Says No* (Vintage Canada, 2003), 9.

46. Michael Pollan, *In Defense of Food: An Eater's Manifesto* (Penguin, 2008), 148.

47. Doc Lew Childre, and Howard Martin, *The HeartMath Solution* (HarperOne, 2001), 89.

48. William Killgore, Ellen Kahn-Greene, Erica Lipizzi, Rachel Newman, Gary Kamimori, and Thomas Balkin, "Sleep Deprivation Reduces Perceived Emotional Intelligence and Constructive Thinking Skills," Sleep Medicine 9 (2008): 517–26.

49. Travis Bradberry, "Multitasking Damages Your Brain and Career, New Studies Suggest," *Forbes*, October 8, 2014, http://www.forbes.com/sites/travisbradberry/2014/10/08/multi-tasking-damages-your-brain-and-career-new-studies-suggest/.

50. Erica Kenney, et al. Prevalence of Inadequate Hydration Among US Children and Disparities by Gender and Race/Ethnicity: National Health and Nutrition Examination Survey, 2009-2012, *American Journal of Public Health*, 2015; 105(8) e113–e118.

51. Mbella Sango, *Sophia's Fire*, (G&V Publishing, Inc., 2005), 30.

52. Abraham Maslow, *Motivation and Personality* (Harper and Row, 1954), 91.

53. Abraham Maslow, *Toward a Psychology of Being* (John Wiley & Sons, 1999), 6.

54. Henry David Thoreau, *Walden* (A Public Domain Book, 2012), Kindle Edition, 21.

55. Bronnie Ware, *The Top Five Regrets of the Dying: A Life Transformed by the Dearly Departing* (Hay House, 2012), Kindle Edition, 214.

56. Ibid., 213.

57. Jeanne E Arnold, et al., *Life at Home in the Twenty-First Century: 32 Families Open Their Doors*, (The Cotsen Institute of Archaelogy Press, 2012), 26.

58. Kiecolt-Glaser, J.K., Loving, T.J., Stowell, J.R., Malarkey, W.B., Lemeshow, S., Dickinson, S.L., et al, Hostile marital interactions, proinflammatory cytokine production, and wound healing, Archives of General Psychiatry (2005), 62(12), 1377–84.

59. Tom Rath, *Vital Friends: The People You Can't Afford to Live Without* (Gallup Press, 2006), 23–24.

60. Robert Louis Stevenson, *The Novels and Tales of Robert Louis Stevenson: An inland voyage. Travels with a donkey*, Edinburgh (Charles Scribner's Sons, 1895), 17.

61. Sami Yenigun, "Play Doesn't End With Childhood: Why Adults Need Recess Too," NPR (August 6, 2014), Web (May 21, 2015), http://www.npr.org/sections/ed/2014/08/06/336360521/play-doesnt-end-with-childhood-why-adults-need-recess-too.

62. Stuart Brown, MD, and Christopher Vaughan, *Play: How It Shapes the Brain, Opens the Imagination, and Invigorates the Soul* (Penguin Publishing Group, 2009), Kindle Edition, 6.

63. Ibid., 4–5.

64. Ibid., 11–12.

65. Ibid., 37.

66. Bernie Siegel, (August 5, 2013), View Your Life as an Experiment, Retrieved from http://berniesiegelmd.com/2013/08/view-your-life-as-an-experiment/.

67. Gabrielle Roth, *Maps to Ecstasy*, (New World Library, 1998), 178.

68. Eckhart Tolle, *A New Earth: Awakening to Your Life Purpose* (Penguin, 2005), 109.

69. Clarissa Pinkola Estés, *Women Who Run with the Wolves* (Ballantine Books, 1992), 299.

70. Charles Eisenstein, *The Yoga of Eating: Transcending Diets and Dogma to Nourish the Natural Self* (New Trends Publishing, 2003), 4–5.

71. Phillippa Lally, Cornelia H. M. van Jaarsveld, Henry W. W. Potts and Jane Wardle, "How are habits formed: Modelling habit formation in the real world" European Journal of Social Psychology, Vol 40, Iss 6, pp 998–1009, October 2010.

72. Robert Kegan and Lisa Laskow Lahey, *How the Way We Talk Can Change the Way We Work* (Jossey-Bass, 2001), 47.

73. Ibid., 63.

74. Ibid., 59.

75. Ibid., 58.

76. *Berkman LF, Syme SL,* "Social networks, host resistance, and mortality: a nine-year fol-low-up study of Alameda County residents," Am J Epidemiol. 1979 Feb; 109(2):186-204.

77. "Strengthen relationships for longer, healthier life," Harvard Health Publications *Healthbeat,* accessed October 2015, http://www.health.harvard.edu/healthbeat/strength-en-relationships-for-longer-healthier-life.

78. Sharrita Forest, "Social support critical to women's weight-loss efforts, study finds," Illinois News Bureau, accessed Oct 2015, https://news.illinois.edu/blog/view/6367/204477.

79. Kevin Helliker, "The Power of a Gentle Nudge: Phone Calls, Even Voice Recordings, Can Get People to Go to the Gym," *The Wall Street Journal* (May 18, 2010), accessed Oct 2015,

80. Lloyd Dean and James Doty, MD, "The Healing Power of Kindness," *Huffington Post,* posted 11/16/2014, as seen on 7/25/15 http://www.huffingtonpost.com/project-compas-sion-stanford/the-healing-power-of-kindness_b_6136272.html.

81. Stuart Davis, *Stuart Davis,* Dharma Pop, 2001, MP3.

82. Nelson Mandela, *Notes to the Future: Words of Wisdom* (Simon and Schuster, 2012), 84.

83. John O'Donohue, *Eternal Echoes: Celtic Reflections on Our Yearning to Belong* (Cliff Street Books/HarperPerennial, 2000), 62.

84 Etienne and Beverly Wenger-Trayner, "Communities of Practice: A Brief Introduction," April 2013, http://wenger-trayner.com/wp-content/uploads/2015/04/07-Brief-introduc-tion-to-communities-of-practice.pdf.

85. Tom Rath and Jim Harter, *Wellbeing: The Five Essential Elements* (Gallup Press, 2010), Kindle Edition, 843–48.

86. Adrienne Rich, *Later Poems: Selected and New 1971–2012* (W.W. Norton, 2013), 128.

87. Brené Brown, *The Gifts of Imperfection: Let Go of Who You Think You're Supposed to Be and Embrace Who You Are* (Hazelden Publishing, 2010), Kindle Edition, 10.

88. Brené Brown, *Daring Greatly: How the Courage to Be Vulnerable Transforms the Way We Live, Love, Parent, and Lead* (Penguin Publishing Group, 2012), Kindle Edition, 75.

89. Bill Plotkin, *Nature and the Human Soul* (New World Library, 2010), 376.

90. Fritof Capra, *The Web of Life* (First Anchor Books, 1996), 96.

91. Ibid., 6–7.

92. Ibid., 37.

93. Joseph Campbell and Bill Moyers, *The Power of Myth* (Knopf DoubleDay Publishing Group, 2011), 183.

94. Larry Dossey, *Space, Time & Medicine*, (Shambhala Publications, 1982), 112.

95. Lisa Wimberger, *Neurosculpting: A Whole-Brain Approach to Heal Trauma, Rewrite Limiting Beliefs, and Find Wholeness* (Sounds True, 2015), 183.